A SAFE PLACE

A SAFE PLACE

A Journal for Women with Breast Cancer

Jennifer Pike

*For my sister, Judy Rose, my father, Geoffrey Pike, and my friends Julie Gibson,
Sylvia Rose, Sally Petitpierre, Ann Gilbert Hopkins, Lucy Stewart, Andrea Maitland,
Sandra Hargreaves, and Stephanie Newsome, all of whom kept my head
above water. And with enormous gratitude also to
Larry Chan and Joyce Frazee.*

– J.P.

First published in 1997 by

Raincoast Books
8680 Cambie Street, Vancouver, B.C., v6p 6m9
(604) 323-7100

CANADIAN CATALOGUING IN PUBLICATION DATA

Pike, Jennifer, 1955-
A safe place

Includes bibliographical references.
ISBN 1-55192-108-1

1. Breast – Cancer – Patients.
2. Breast – Cancer – Psychological aspects.
3. Diaries (Blank-books). I. Title.

RC280.B8P54 1997   616.99'449   C97-910400-9

Grateful acknowledgment is made to the following for permission to reprint previously published material:

Extract from *The Alchemy of Illness* by
Kat Duff, copyright © 1993 by Kat Duff.
Reprinted by permission of Random House.

Extract from *The Artist's Way: A Spiritual
Path to Higher Creativity*, copyright © 1992
by Julia Cameron. Reprinted by permission
of Jeremy P. Tarcher, Inc., The Putnam
Publishing Group.

Extract from "Encounters with Patients"
from *Head First: The Biology of Hope and the
Healing Power of the Human Spirit* by
Norman Cousins, copyright © 1989 by
Norman Cousins. Reprinted by permission
of Dutton/Signet-Penguin USA.

Extract from *Grace and Grit: Spirituality
and Healing in the Life and Death of Treya
Killam Wilber* by Ken Wilber, copyright
© 1991 by Ken Wilber. Reprinted by
permission of Shambhala Publications.

"Late Fragment" from *A New Path to the
Waterfall* by Raymond Carver, copyright
© 1989 by the estate of Raymond Carver.
Reprinted by permission of Grove/Atlantic.

Quotations from *Spinning Straw into
Gold: Your Emotional Recovery from Breast
Cancer* by Ronnie Kaye, copyright © 1991 by
Lamppost Press and Ronnie Kaye. Reprinted
by permission of Simon and Schuster.

PRINTED AND BOUND IN CANADA

CONTENTS

ACKNOWLEDGMENTS

THE HELP OF THE FOLLOWING is gratefully acknowledged: All the women who generously agreed to be interviewed for this book; and J. T. Sandy, M.D., F.R.C.S.(C), clinical professor emeritus of surgery, University of British Columbia; Elaine Drysdale, M.D., F.R.C.P.(C), clinical associate professor, Faculty of Medicine, University of British Columbia, and consultant psychiatrist, B.C. Cancer Agency; A. W. Tolcher, M.D., B.C. Cancer Agency; Lawrence Chan, D.C., N.D.; B. Ann Hilton, R.N., Ph.D., associate professor, School of Nursing, University of British Columbia; Elizabeth Dohan, M.S.W., B.C. Cancer Agency; Lenore Nicholson, R.N.; Silvia Wilson, R.N., B.Sc.N., M.N.; David Noble, head librarian, B.C. Cancer Agency; Anna Daly; Jennifer Bradbury; B.C. and Yukon Breast Cancer Information Project; Ivo Olivotto, M.D., F.R.C.P.(C), chair, Breast Cancer Tumor Group, B.C. Cancer Agency.

INTRODUCTION

Believing that there is a power that can make you well – whether that's
God, or your surgeon, or your own will – can help you to get well. . . .
History is full of accounts of miracles, and while we have no
laboratory proof that these accounts are accurate, there
are simply too many of them to dismiss.
  – Dr. Susan Love's Breast Book

It's not the end of the world. There's no need to be so frightened.
  – Adine, diagnosed 1971

WHEN I WAS TOLD I had breast cancer on April Fools' Day 1993 (a peculiarly appropriate date, I thought, even at the time), I remember being overwhelmed by fear, anger, incredulity, and shock. Information and well-meaning advice were showered upon me until I was so panicked I simply didn't know what to do next. My brain certainly couldn't process everything, so I turned to writing it all down. From then on the lined yellow pad of paper I found in the drawer became my sounding board and confessional.

My feelings were probably less than admirable, and I didn't think I could tell anyone else about them, but the act of putting them on a piece of paper helped to give me some perspective and to distance myself from the horror. My whole world seemed to be disintegrating; all the things I had taken for granted for so long had turned out to be false, an illusion. My health, for a start. In my fool's paradise I assumed, although I didn't think about it much, that I would live out a normal life span. I believed that I would only have to consider the prospect of death when I reached an age more appropriate for such thoughts than 47. The cancer diagnosis changed all of that. I was forcibly reminded that I wasn't going to live forever.

That lined yellow pad of paper turned into a journal of feelings and observations that I wrote down almost every day – sometimes just a paragraph, sometimes a few pages – as I went through surgery, chemotherapy, and radiation. It was a shoulder to cry on and a repository for my anger and fear. The act of writing enabled me to find enough strength to continue with all the information-gathering and filtering you have to do when you are diagnosed with cancer, and it also clarified the decision-making process for me.

Painful as it now is to look at the journal, I am glad I have it. My journal shows me how far I have come, and it also reminds me of how kind and compassionate people were – family, friends, and even complete strangers. It reminds me, too, that breast cancer isn't necessarily a fatal disease: people *do* survive it. Parts of my journal are included in this book.

Now it is your turn. Presumably you are reading this because you have, or someone you are close to has, breast cancer. You may also be wondering if writing about the experience will help. I hope it will.

The purpose of the journal is to provide emotional support. Although everyone reacts differently, there do seem to be common experiences as women go through the various stages of breast cancer: diagnosis, making treatment decisions, treatment itself, and how women feel afterward.

This journal isn't intended in any way to be a substitute for professional therapy. Call it do-it-yourself life support, if you like, or emotional first aid, a companion, or just a safe place for you to write whatever you want in complete privacy. It deals only peripherally with the medical aspects of the disease, although there will be hints on how to cope with treatment as you go through it, as well as quotations from women, like me, who have been through it before you. You will also find quotations from other writers and health practitioners, along with some affirmations and prompts to help you to start writing about your own experiences and feelings. It will always be a place for you to answer the question, "How do I really feel?"

You will probably discover your own affirmations as you go along; everyone deals with illness in their own way, and sometimes a certain repeated phrase can help displace some of the negative noise that closes down our minds at stressful times. Many women find relaxation and visualization techniques helpful, too; some are suggested here, although you will undoubtedly create your own. Because there are as many ways of dealing with feelings about cancer as there are people who have it, not all of the journal will be relevant to your own circumstances. Just skip the parts that aren't useful to you and concentrate on what you can use. There will be blank pages for you to write and draw on if you feel so inclined. There will also be pages for recording your dreams, as many people find it helpful to understand them.

Even though you may feel alone, don't imagine you are the only person who has ever had to go through the distressing and alarming experience of having breast cancer. There are lots of us living with the disease: you have probably already heard that one in nine women in Canada will develop breast cancer in her lifetime. And there are more mind-boggling statistics: Nearly 18,600 new cases of breast cancer occurred in Canada in 1996 alone. In the United States newly diagnosed cases of breast cancer total nearly 200,000 each year. It is estimated that there are two million women in North America living with breast cancer.

At the end of this book there is a list of publications that may be helpful to you, too. It isn't an exhaustive list; there have been many books written about cancer and breast cancer in particular, and I am sure there will be more. Most are available from bookstores or libraries. If you are interested in more reading material, you can always ask your doctors what books they recommend. Many women find they want to read as much as they can, so that they are well informed when it comes to investigating their options. Others choose not to know as much – they would rather just get on with treatment and the rest of their lives. Do whatever is right for you.

ABOUT WRITING A JOURNAL

I did keep a journal. The very fact of keeping a journal was helpful. You can talk to yourself about your illness, and that's helpful with any distressing situation. If you can put it down on paper,
it becomes less intimidating.
– Joan A, diagnosed 1986, mother of two

I'd read that keeping a journal is supposed to be really beneficial for your mental health, but time . . . who's got the time?
– Debbie, diagnosed 1995, mother of two

I SUPPOSE IF WE sat down and thought about it, hardly any of us would ever find the time to keep a journal. Most of us lead busy lives and tend to put our own needs last.

A diary, however, can be a powerful tool. Virginia Woolf tells us that she wrote her diaries to bring order out of chaos. Few of us can write as well as she did, but she was right. You have been diagnosed with cancer; you can't change that, but you can do something to make it less stressful. By recording what is happening to you and your feelings about it, you allow stress and fear to come out into the open instead of having it churn inside you. You may then find some constructive energy to do what has to be done.

Remember that you are not writing for an audience. You don't have to consider anyone else's feelings, and you can write in any fashion you want. No one will be checking your spelling or grammar, and there is no right or wrong way to write a journal. You don't have to worry about style, and you can be tidy or messy. Feel free to tell your inner censor or critic – or whatever you call that disapproving persona that sometimes takes over – to take a hike while you are writing. You may contradict yourself from day to day. It doesn't matter: there can be many different, yet valid, perspectives on any subject, and with a subject such as breast cancer you are probably being flooded with confusing messages, anyway. Writing it all down will help you to synthesize that information and will also enable you to make the decisions that are right for you with greater confidence.

It is important that you write when you feel like writing. Be spontaneous, write fast, don't edit yourself too much. You probably have to edit yourself in your relationships with other people, so your diary is the one place your real self can be displayed, warts and all. This is the place where you can say angry things to the people around you without hurting them. In other words, it is the place to let off steam if that is what you feel like doing. Or you can use the diary for quiet reflection. It is entirely up to you.

If you find that you have writer's block, try writing with your other hand. Sometimes that will be enough to get you started. Or you can try referring to yourself in the third person, using "she" instead of "I."

You may discover in yourself a desire to go on writing a daily journal once you have completed this one. People don't just write diaries when they are in pain or unhappy. As a nonjudgmental listener a diary can help make sense of life and can also serve as a useful reference point for those times when you want to look back.

Because it will undoubtedly include material that is painful, you may not want to reread your journal after your course of treatment is complete. I still find my own journal quite difficult to reread because it is so full of anger and pain, but when I finally looked at and understood my feelings and dreams, I realized that the experience of having cancer was by no means entirely negative. I was reminded of the love and affection that surrounded me, and of my love for the landscape of British Columbia. Each of these things played a crucial role in my recovery.

How are you really feeling right now?

AFTER THE DIAGNOSIS

The first thing a woman thinks of when diagnosed
with breast cancer is: "Will I die?"
– Dr. Susan Love's Breast Book

Cancer is not some kind of death sentence at all. It has always been a chronic challenge that you take on, but seldom THIS IS IT. The word *cancer* itself is so frightening. Even when the prognosis is good, it kind of numbs the person. It assaults every sense you have. We are stuck on the sadder stories and we don't advertise the successes.

– Silvia Wilson, former oncology nurse and daughter of a woman diagnosed with breast cancer in 1995

I REMEMBER that my own first feelings after diagnosis were of anger and disbelief. I was driving to work after having had an ultrasound test (a diagnostic tool that uses sound waves to view your body) during which the radiologist had shown me a tiny but unmistakably solid lump on the screen. I had to wait 24 hours for the pathology report, and I was screaming in the car, "I can't have cancer. I won't have cancer!" Because, of course, what you hear when you receive a diagnosis of breast cancer *is* a death sentence. The Big C. But one of the things I have discovered throughout my own experience and in the course of researching this book is that although breast cancer is a chronic disease, it isn't necessarily fatal. Many women live for years after diagnosis and treatment, dying at a ripe old age of something else entirely.

One day while I was visiting Michael, a friend who was in the final stages of AIDS, he suddenly said, "I wish I just had cancer." Up to that moment I hadn't considered myself to be particularly lucky, but I understood him: at least I had a chance.

How did you receive your diagnosis? Was it from your physician, the surgeon, or someone else? Was it given to you in person, or over the telephone? Did you "know" you had cancer before you were actually diagnosed? Did you have to convince the doctors that something was wrong? I have talked to many women who say they knew that something was wrong even when their mammograms or biopsies showed nothing abnormal. Many women have said they had to work hard to convince their doctors to check further.

I felt quite calm after the diagnosis. I'm a nurse and I work with AIDS patients, and I see the devastation they go through, and I said to myself once that if I ever have to have something big happen to me, I would rather have breast cancer than anything else. So I wasn't that surprised.

— *Lynda, diagnosed 1994*

I ASKED EACH of the women I interviewed for this book what one important thing they would tell a woman who was just diagnosed. Here are some of their replies:

"It's a hell of a way to join a club, but you are in the company of some wonderful women out there. Find the strength, because you have to in order to keep going. It's amazing how and where you find it, but you do."

    – Jo, diagnosed 1982

"My advice to someone newly diagnosed is this: you don't have to do anything you don't feel good about. The thing to do is to learn as much as you can, and talk to as many people as you can who've had similar experiences. And always ask questions. Never feel you shouldn't ask a question because it's a silly question. Be as informed as humanly possible and set yourself some things you plan to do in the future. Assume that you are going to recover your full health and that these things are going to be possible. Also, take people into your confidence. Don't hide the situation."

    – Joan A

"A lot of other women are in exactly the same situation as you are. There is an end to all this treatment. Initially that's what looked so onerous to me – the length of the chemo and radiation and everything. At first you're feeling quite good and surgery is no big deal, but as you progressively go through treatment, you feel shittier and shittier. There will be an end to it, and it's so nice when you reach it. It's such a big milestone to have gotten to the end of it."

    – Debbie

"You'll come out six months later, or whenever treatment ends, with a way better outlook than you thought you would. Amazingly, things will return to a semblance of normality. The other thing is to take it one step at a time."

    – Angie, diagnosed 1994

"Don't make hard and fast decisions not to have a mastectomy instead of a lumpectomy. Don't be so worried about mastectomy. Have someone talk through body-image issues with you. If you have a good self-concept and your ego isn't so tied up in how you look, you will do way better."

    – Brenda, diagnosed 1983 and 1993

"Take control. Define for yourself what you want to know."

    – Elaine, diagnosed 1995

"Have faith that you're going to be okay. Just believe. It's a rough road to go through, and going through chemo, you do have your doubts."

    – Joan D, diagnosed 1995

MOST PEOPLE HAVE FEELINGS that run the gamut from anger, fear, denial, guilt, shock, and depression, to secret relief that there really is something wrong with them. Like Lynda, quoted earlier, some women are calm about the diagnosis, as if it were expected. I was convinced for a long time that they had mixed my test results up with someone else's – I guess that was denial.

I called a friend, Carol, who was diagnosed in 1991, after I got my diagnosis, and told her about how my emotions were all over the place. She said briskly: "Perfectly normal, my dear." And indeed it is. You are not crazy. Carol went on to say, "Don't worry about it. Look after yourself. That's the most important thing. And you must *want* to be well." Most people reach some kind of equilibrium or achieve some form of acceptance after going through the emotional storms, although you quite often oscillate between relative calm and the more extreme feelings.

Describe how you felt when you first received the diagnosis of cancer.

Reactions to diagnosis are as broad as the breadth of personalities I see. Some people are placid, with no overt reaction, others are anxious and react as they would to anything else: as threatened. I'm not sure that stoic people who don't show much don't suffer more.

– *Dr. J. T. Sandy, surgeon*

AS I MENTIONED EARLIER, I was very angry when I got the diagnosis. I thought I had been doing everything right: exercising regularly, eating a healthy diet, not smoking. It didn't seem fair. Well, it isn't fair that anyone gets cancer, and there is nothing fair about the arbitrariness of who gets it and who doesn't, so it is up to you to work out a way of coping with it. You may feel that, because you don't want to be a cancer patient at all, each new piece of information you get admits you further into a world you would rather know nothing about. News flash: you don't have to be patient if you don't want to be. Fight. Use the energy that your anger gives you to fight for your health.

Perhaps you aren't angry at all. You may be sad or tired, or you may just want to get on with getting well again. How do you really feel? See what your feelings look like on paper. They are yours. You have every right to them. Does writing them down help to put them in perspective?

Your anger will save you.

— *Margarethe Kahn,*
psychologist

*I will use my anger to help
me fight this disease.*

You have had the diagnosis. So remember that the worst has already happened. Try not to go over it time and time again in your mind. You are probably feeling as anxious as you will ever be about anything. You have every reason to feel this way. Uncertainty goes along with a breast cancer diagnosis because those of us who have had it will never know for sure if it will come back. But there are ways of coping with anxiety: relaxation techniques, support groups, and counseling. If you can possibly do it, try to put aside your worries about death and dying. Right now you need all of your energy to cope with what is going on around you, and to deal with treatment. You will be able to deal with your own mortality later when you can concentrate on such issues more fully.

How are you feeling right now? What makes you afraid? What makes you happy?

I can choose to think more cheerful
thoughts, and I can fight the fear.

"I was in the abyss the first week after diagnosis before treatment. I woke up in the middle of the night feeling I was alone and maybe dying and trying to comprehend dying. I realized I was fine at that moment, staring at the ceiling, saying, 'I'm fine. I'm not dying at this moment. If I go one day at a time, everything will be fine. I can cope with one day at a time. I will be alive and not dying if I just do one day at a time.' I used that a lot."

    – Judy, diagnosed 1992

"Don't look 10 years down the road. Don't even look a week down the road at all the things you have to go through. Just try to get through this step."

    – Angie

"Every now and then this little voice pipes up inside me: 'This isn't going to get me. I won't let it.'"

    – from my own journal, April 1993

"There are many different reactions to cancer: some people are just blasé and say, 'So it's breast cancer and, of course, I'm going to have treatment and then be fine.' Then there are others who are totally off the wall, who can't think, can't hear anything you say. It's a whole spectrum. Being blasé is a way of coping, the same way denial is a way of coping. You can deny or be blasé until you're ready to think about things and deal with it. Take advantage of everything: support groups, one-on-one counseling, all the education things that are available. Be really open and ask questions. To be involved is one of the best ways to be involved in your own care. Be in the driver's seat rather than have someone else telling you what to do."

    – Lenore Nicholson, oncology nurse

THERE ARE NO RULES about who gets cancer and who doesn't. Good health seems arbitrary: "I live right. How come I'm sick? You live wrong. How come you're not sick?" Despite what the newspapers say, no one knows for sure yet why some people get cancer and others don't. The greatest risk factor of all for getting breast cancer is the fact that you are a woman. Fewer than one percent of breast cancers are diagnosed in men.

What were your reactions to getting cancer?

I talked about it right from the first biopsy. I decided I was not going to remain silent about why I was off work. I'm not doing any woman a service by remaining silent.

– *Elaine*

THERE IS ANOTHER REASON to write a journal. Sometimes you can't talk freely to the people closest to you because they are just that – too close for you to be able to talk about your emotions. If for some reason you are coping with the diagnosis on your own, without support, that is another reason to write. And remember that you may make friends along the way as you go through treatment; a kind of wartime camaraderie can develop with people who are in the same situation as you are.

Have you told your family about the diagnosis? How did you tell them? How did they react? If you have children, how should you tell them? Or did you tell them? What about your friends? If you have a partner, what did he or she do? How did you feel about it?

We told the kids quite straightforwardly. We never pretended about things with them. There was no hiding from the fact that I was having treatment – it was better that they knew. My 11-year-old knew there was a chance I might not recover. My husband was devastated. We went for a walk after we got home, and when we were in the store, he just broke down in tears. He felt he couldn't cope or manage the children on his own if I didn't recover . . . but he was very supportive a lot of the time. I think he felt very threatened by it, and I found him hard to deal with at times.

– *Joan A*

I find myself playing a
game on the bus: won-
dering who among the
other people has cancer.
In the hospital waiting
room I try to guess
who's the patient
in each group.
– from my own diary,
May 1993

IT SEEMS INCONCEIVABLE that life can go on around you while you are suffering through your own version of the tortures of the damned. You may find yourself resenting people who don't have cancer, and those people could be part of your own family. Here are what some other women felt:

"I never resented my partner for being healthy. He was listening to me and trying to reassure me. Being positive."
  – Judy

"Some women with young children wonder, Will I be here to raise them?"
  – Elizabeth Dohan, oncology social worker

"I have two kids: five and seven years old. The seven-year-old is a serious little boy. He wants to be a scientist when he grows up and wants all the details about everything, so I did tell him exactly how cancer works. There was a support group for kids run by the Cancer Agency, put on by the music and art therapist, so I put him in that program, and it helped. With my five-year-old I tried to broach the subject, but he couldn't have cared less. He just walked away. I found that really difficult. I wanted him to know there were going to be things happening, but it all went over the top of his head."
  – Debbie

"My daughters were 20 and 22 and very concerned about their risks. My son was 15 and very worried. He communicated with his friends and told his girlfriends they should be doing BSE [breast self-examination]. My husband was right there if I needed things. He enjoyed being needed. The kids were impressed at how he could cope. He put the garbage out for the first time in 10 years! He was quite self-absorbed and got on with his own stuff if I didn't ask for help. They don't know automatically. I found it better to take the initiative. It was useful to be in control and able to tell people if I needed help."
  – Brenda

"I think it's difficult for men for several reasons. First of all, men aren't socialized to talk about their feelings, so they don't do it naturally the way women do. They often feel awkward in showing emotions. Secondly, they usually don't have a readily available support system to the same extent as women. When a woman is upset, she can cry and then phone a girlfriend who will listen to her distress. When a man is upset, he is more likely to hide his feelings. Even if he does express his feelings more openly, he may find that his friends don't know how to respond. . . . Men are less likely to ask, 'Jack, how are you really feeling?'. . . The third cause for difficulty is that the man often feels that his distress is of little importance relative to the distress of his partner, who may be frightened for her own survival and who may be feeling unwell due to treatment. Thus men's feelings can get lost in the shuffle. Yet it should be noted that the husband can be undergoing a tremendous amount of stress. . . . There should be more support, including support groups, for such individuals, but the attention tends to be directed to the people who actually have the cancer."

– Dr. Elaine Drysdale, psychiatrist

What has been your experience with family and friends? Or are you coping by yourself?

Day 7 [after diagnosis]: Woke at 5:00 a.m. with the usual terror and brain overdrive. So much to do. Have the urge to tidy up my affairs and the apartment before going into surgery. Hard to concentrate. Saw the lawyer about making a will – have divided my vast estate between my brother and sister. Now the hot tap in the bathroom isn't working. I can't deal with all this stuff.
– from my own diary, April 1993

I DISCOVERED LATER that an urge to tidy the closets is a fairly common reaction, as is the inability to concentrate on anything other than the task immediately at hand, which is usually how to deal with all this arcane information about cancer that you are getting whether you want it or not. Having a cancer diagnosis puts you into a bizarre twilight for a while, a kind of underworld of which you were probably not conscious before. Each piece of information you get admits you further into this world in which you don't want to be, so I guess it is natural for the mind to seize upon something domestically ordinary and achievable in the face of an avalanche of fear-provoking half-information. Embarking upon a flurry of spring cleaning can be constructive as well as good exercise.

You may worry, as I did, that you haven't made a will. Perhaps you need to appoint someone to take care of the children should anything happen to you, or there may be some family business that needs to be sorted out. How are you coping?

ONE THING I REMEMBER CLEARLY is the feeling of not being able to take a really deep breath because of the anxiety in my throat and stomach. A friend then taught me some yoga-breathing techniques that gave me some respite. I tried to do them at least once a day. There are several good books on yoga, and there are yoga classes available in most communities. Check your local newspaper or community center. You might want to record your own ideas and thoughts on relaxation techniques.

Relaxation Exercise:
Close your eyes and take
several deep breaths, letting the breath in and
out slowly, feeling how
the breath changes in
your nostrils as you
breathe in and out. Cry, if
you want to. Some peo-
ple think tears help to
free up emotions and
cleanse the body of tox-
ins. If there are sounds
that distract you, don't
try to push them away,
just notice them and set
them aside while you are
breathing.

*I will deal with this one step at a time. I
will remember to breathe deeply.*

... the theory that inse-
cure, self-critical people
who put the needs of
others before their own
are prone to the disease
strikes me as nonsense.
There are an awful lot of
insecure, self-critical
people I know who do
not have cancer.

— *Joyce Wadler*, My Breast

YOU MAY HAVE BEEN feeling that you somehow caused the cancer, that it is your fault that you have it. You may also be aware of all the theories about a "cancer personality" – theories that are completely unproven, incidentally. Some writers have succeeded in laying guilt at the door of the sufferer, as if she doesn't have enough to worry about.

Because I have a strong opinion on this, here is mine: *It is not your fault. You did not cause the cancer.* Nobody knows yet what causes breast cancer in any more than the tiny percentage of women who have a strong family history of it and carry the gene. And you did not get cancer because you are a terrible person or even a semi-terrible person. Think about how many less than admirable people are walking around out there who don't have cancer.

As Dr. A.W. Tolcher, a medical oncologist, puts it: "There are five to seven genetic mutations required to form cancer. That's why breast cancer happens after a period of time – it can be from exposure to a lot of different things. Finding one smoking gun is next to impossible. People should not look at their lives hunting for responsibility from things they did. An accumulation of mutations led to this. Don't dissect it. It takes away from looking at the future."

What are your feelings about why you got cancer?

I tell people that there are many factors involved in the development of cancer. Cancer is a collection of abnormal cells that have developed for a number of reasons. The body is constantly making new cells by a process where each cell duplicates its information and then divides to create a new cell. It might be helpful to compare the body's functioning to that of a Xeroxing machine: we have a cell, and then we make a copy of that cell. At some point the machine can produce a flawed copy, due to a number of reasons. Normally the immune system in the body recognizes the flawed copy and destroys it. . . . Unfortunately sometimes the bad copy is not noticed and remains to be recopied later, resulting in a whole batch of bad copies.

A tumor is a batch of bad
copies. We can look at the
causes of cancer from
two perspectives. First,
we can examine what
caused the flawed copies
to occur in the first
place. . . . For example,
there may be genetic fac-
tors, environmental fac-
tors, such as exposure to
radiation or pesticides, or
dietary factors. From a
second perspective, we
can focus on the functioning of the immune
system and the factors
that affect it, including
medications, stress, and
emotions. Most cancer
research has traditionally
focused on the causes of
abnormal cell production
(the Xeroxing compo-
nent). In the past decade,
there has been increasing
interest and research
into the role of the
immune system.
— *Dr. Elaine Drysdale*

MANY PEOPLE WONDER about the effect of stress on the immune system. There seems to be evidence that stress does have an effect on the body, so we can do things to strengthen our immune systems, to be more attentive to our bodies. We can try to reduce stress by finding ways to relax or by changing our perspective on life and doing our best to enhance our overall health.

How do you cope with stress?

The relative importance of the immune system may differ for different individuals. Some people might easily create flawed cells, possibly due to genetic factors or due to such overwhelming biological factors as living near highly radioactive material, such as Chernobyl, and thus cancer may develop despite a really well-functioning immune system. Unfortunately people often blame themselves unnecessarily, when perhaps they are facing tremendous biological factors that may still be unknown. . . . I sometimes say to people who think they got ill because they were not spiritual enough, "Look at the story of Job in the Old Testament. He was a very good man, yet all of these troubles befell him, anyway. The rain falls on the good and the bad alike."
– *Dr. Elaine Drysdale*

DOZENS OF PEOPLE (not people with cancer) told me that I should have and maintain a "positive" attitude, and that being positive would make me well. This assertion left me with the unspoken conclusion that if I wasn't positive all the time it would be my fault if I didn't get well. I found myself becoming profoundly irritated; if I couldn't tell anyone how I really felt about having breast cancer, I would be shutting those feelings away without acknowledging them. You can't feel positive all day, every day, play Pollyanna, or try to fulfill someone else's expectations of what you should be feeling if you are actually angry, frightened, or depressed. And even if you could, it wouldn't prevent you from having cancer.

David Spiegel, M.D., author of *Living Beyond Limits: New Hope and Help for Facing Life-Threatening Illness*, refers to this as "the prison of positive thinking. The last thing you need is to feel bad about feeling bad."

How do *you* really feel?

If you talk about having a
"fighting spirit" rather
than being "positive,"
you can be yourself and
be proactive.
— *Elizabeth Dohan*

Overall, it's probably better to be thinking more optimistically than it is to think negatively and cynically about everything. But that's something that you have to work through. You can come to that stage after you've worked through all the anger and frustration. After you have dealt with that, hopefully you'll come out the other side and be able to go on with some sense of greater serenity and peacefulness and optimism. But you can't just paint positive thinking on like makeup.

– Dr. Elaine Drysdale

I need the support of women who've had this and I find it really helpful
just to be there at the support group I've been going to for three months.
I wish they were held every two weeks instead of once a month. The first
one I went to, there was a total of five of us women who had five-year-
olds. You sort of feel that you're only 39 and it can't happen to that
many women your age, and then you see other women younger than
yourself and you think, God, this is a wicked disease. This is not fair.

– Debbie

MANY WOMEN FIND that it is of the greatest help to talk to someone who has been through the same experience. It can also help to make you feel less alone. Many attend support groups while others find someone who can help them one-on-one.

I am almost ashamed to admit that I had to overcome a lifelong reluctance to becoming a "joiner" before I could bring myself to attend a support group. I had read as much as I could and had talked to various women one at a time. The first group I went to was for newly diagnosed women, as well as for those who were going through chemotherapy and radiation.

I could hardly move my right arm after surgery and was convinced that the arm would never be normal again, but then a woman in the group whipped open her blouse and showed me how well her armpit had healed in the two years since her first surgery. It looked completely normal. I will always be grateful to her for that.

It was a huge relief to find that other women had the same feelings and experiences, and that I was free to talk about mine. One woman there referred to support groups as "love among strangers." Another said, "You can't swallow your feelings. You get clarity when you talk to someone else." That is exactly what it has been like in the several groups I have been to since diagnosis.

Many cities and towns now have breast cancer support groups. Ask your physician or the local cancer society if there is one near you. Some districts also have volunteer visitor programs where a woman who has had a similar experience to yours will come to see you, or phone you, and you will be able to talk about your concerns with her. A list of these organizations, along with a list of books and other publications, can be found at the end of this book.

Some women react to their diagnosis by wanting to read everything they can about breast cancer and the issues surrounding it. These women find that a better understanding of the disease and its treatment empowers them to ask more informed questions and gives them a greater sense of control as they progress through a difficult time. Others choose a less activist approach, such as reading a little, not asking many questions, accepting treatment recommendations from the physicians; in short, just getting on with it.

Whichever path feels right for you is the one you should take. My own experience was that I could get the doctors to answer my questions if I knew the right ones to ask, which, of course, I did not until I had done some research. *Dr. Susan Love's Breast Book* was my mentor after diagnosis, and Bernie Siegel's *Love, Medicine and Miracles* was my emotional support. A wonderful new booklet called *What You Need to Know About Breast Cancer* – available free from the various Breast Cancer Information Exchange Projects (see Breast Cancer Information Projects in "Other Resources" for contact information) – is written by survivors of breast cancer and is intended for newly diagnosed women. I wish it had been available when I was diagnosed. Further on in this journal you will find some suggested questions for you to ask at the different stages of your treatment.

You might want to note some of your own experiences in support groups, make a list of your own reading, or record useful quotations culled from what you have read.

The thought of dying
never occurred to me. It
wasn't until I was going
to the support group and
reading that I realized
people do think they're
going to die. I wouldn't
allow myself to think of
that. I didn't want to read
during treatment because
I didn't want to think.

– *Lynda*

I dabbled a bit in visualization to deal with the fluid in my arm [lymphedema], and at the same time envisioned an outline, a typical stickman: head, shoulders, trunk, arms, legs. I envisioned a very bright white line all around this body, and flashing across the upper chest in red is a neon sign that says CANCER-FREE ZONE.

– *Elaine*

PERHAPS GETTING THE DIAGNOSIS has made it difficult for you to get a good night's sleep. If you are not usually a pill popper, you may be reluctant to ask your doctor for a prescription. However, if you are getting desperate, you should do whatever it takes to make you feel better. If that means taking sleeping pills or an antidepressant, that is fine. It is perfectly all right to seek medical intervention at a time when your emotions have gone haywire.

Other ways of dealing with anxiety are to use relaxation, visualization, and meditation techniques. Audiotapes are also helpful (available from libraries, retail outlets, or through your cancer hospital). Some women make their own relaxation tapes using a soothing voice (their own or a friend's) and music.

A suggested visualization: Find a quiet place where you will not be disturbed. Close your eyes and breathe deeply and regularly until you have established a comfortable rhythm and are feeling relaxed. You may have a favorite place – real or imaginary. Imagine you are in that place. Look at the light and the colors. Notice if there are any special fragrances associated with it. What sounds do you hear? If you are by the water, can you hear the waves? Is the water lapping at the shore? Is the wind rustling the leaves on the trees? Is there music playing? Are there any birds or animals, or other people with you? Immerse yourself in all the sights and sounds and fragrances, and stay there. When you are ready, start to notice your breathing again, how the air feels in your nostrils as you breathe in and out, making you ready to join the world again. Then open your eyes and take a few moments to appreciate how relaxed you feel.

You could also visualize a large, confused cancer cell, and your body's defenses rushing to neutralize it and then flushing the dead cell out and away. Judy, quoted in this book, remembers a social worker talking about how fragile cancer cells really are, and how easily they can be destroyed. This could form another part of your visualization. You could also visualize parts of your body, such as the lymphatic system, normal cells, cancer cells (dead or nearly dead), killer cells, bone marrow, and so on. Draw a picture.

I would visualize peace
and harmony flowing
into my body, and stress
and disease being wiped
out. I still use that
visualization.
— *Lynda*

May my body be strong and healthy.
May my heart be peaceful.

ANOTHER WAY TO get yourself to relax is to lie down, close your eyes and, starting with your toes, tense each part of your body, then let it go and allow it to relax. Pay particular attention to your stomach and diaphragm, then your neck and shoulders – these are the parts that seem to get the most tight.

Write down a meditation or relaxation technique here that works for you so that you can come back and use it again later.

THIS CAN'T BE HAPPENING TO ME . . .

Most of us go through a stage of not believing that this can actually be happening, that there must have been a terrible mistake and that the lab must have mixed up our pathology results with somebody else's. I was well into my treatment before I could fully accept in my heart that I did indeed have cancer. Then I started to contemplate making bargains with God: if you make me better, I promise to be a better person and to lead a better life. . . . I didn't tell anyone else about it, but the thoughts were there nevertheless.

Have you had thoughts like this?

... dream work gives you access to important creative, curative, and renewing aspects of the self that might otherwise go unrecognized.

— *Tristine Rainer,* The New Diary

DREAMS CAN BE a way of releasing pain and stress, and can help you to recognize who and where you are. If you write them down, you can begin to understand what they are telling you. By looking back at what you have written, you will be able to discern patterns and see how far you have come.

At the end of each section of this journal you will find blank pages where you can record your dreams at that particular stage. Some people keep a "dream book" beside the bed while others use a tape recorder and write the dreams down later. Whatever method you use, it is important to record a dream right after you wake. If you wait until later, you are likely to forget crucial parts of the dream. Also, the very act of writing down an emotion-filled dream can help you to recognize and deal with anxiety and fear. There are many helpful books about dreaming, some of which are listed at the end of this book. Counseling can also help you to understand your dreams.

Have your dream patterns changed? Are you dreaming more, or less?

A dream may survive a lifetime of neglect or an onslaught of interpretations and remain an icon and a fertile enigma for years of reflection. The point in working with a dream is never to translate it into a final meaning, but always to give it honor and respect, drawing from it as much meaningfulness and imaginative meditation as possible.

— *Thomas Moore,*
Care of the Soul

TREATMENT DECISIONS

The most important thing is to pick a therapy that you believe in and
proceed with a positive attitude.
– Bernie Siegel, *Love, Medicine and Miracles*

I would say that the ones that want to find out as much as they can about what's going on, and the ones who question, definitely do better at going through treatment.

— *Lenore Nicholson*

JUST ABOUT EVERY WOMAN I have spoken to agrees that making treatment decisions is difficult, but that once you have made them you have to do your utmost to view both your decision as the right one and the treatment as helpful. These decisions often have to be made on the basis of inconclusive information, no matter how many books and articles you may have read. You may also feel that the choices you have to make are from unpalatable alternatives. Most doctors and other health professionals believe that it helps the patient if she takes an active part in the decision-making process about her treatment – it gives her a sense of being in control of events which she may feel are happening much too fast and without any say-so from her. So if you can participate actively in conversations with your doctors and nurses, asking questions if there is anything you don't understand, you may end up feeling better about a lot of things.

Your choice may be between having a mastectomy or lumpectomy, and you might wonder what difference one or the other will make to your chances of survival. If you choose mastectomy, you may be wondering about breast reconstruction afterward and how you will look. (There is a section about reconstructive surgery later on in the journal.) You may wonder what the scar will look like. There is no such thing as a stupid question where cancer is concerned, and you can rehearse the questions you want to ask your surgeon or physician here. You will find suggested questions about surgery and the various treatments available further on in this journal under the heading for each treatment.

Doctors don't have many definitive answers about why we get cancer, but they do have answers about the effectiveness of treatment and about any side effects. Doctors' offices can be intimidating places, and I know from experience that once you are there it is easy to forget the things you meant to ask. So if you write your questions down in this book, take it along to appointments with you. Again, try the reading list at the end of the journal for publications that can help you to prepare the right questions.

Many women like to take a friend or family member along to their medical appointments. My own instinct was to ask someone to go with me each time, and I am so glad that I did. My good friend Julie came to the surgeon's office and to the cancer hospital with me and took notes, which I was appreciative of later because I had forgotten about three-quarters of what I had been told. Most medical professionals like it, too, when the patient takes a friend or family member along for appointments. I understand now why people who work in jobs where they have to be serious use black humor to relieve stress. There is not a whole lot of laughter attached to cancer, as you already know, and we found it a great relief to be able to make bad jokes about it.

Be your own advocate. I had read my hospital admitting form upside down as it was emerging from the printer at the admitting desk and saw, to my horror, that I was booked for a total mastectomy. I knew I was just supposed to be having a lumpectomy, so I refused to sign any hospital form until the surgeon appeared at my bedside that evening and confirmed that someone had indeed put the wrong information on the form. No doubt the hospital bureaucracy could have done without my stubbornness, but I felt better for having stood up for myself (quite apart from not having had to lose a breast unnecessarily), and the experience taught me to question anything I didn't feel comfortable with or didn't understand. Again, it gave me a feeling of being in control of the events that were taking place around me.

The next few pages are for you to list your questions for the surgeon, oncologist, or family doctor, and enough space has been provided for the answers you receive.

Another pair of ears going in with you is helpful for medical appointments. They may hear slightly differently from you. As your anxiety level increases, your ability to hear decreases, and the other person can pick up that information and relay it to you.

– *Silvia Wilson*

Ninety-nine percent of
the time it's good to take
a friend along, but if the
relationship is not good,
or if the other person is
angry or upset, it's not
good, it gets in the
way instead.
– *Lenore Nicholson*

IF YOU ARE ONE of those people who have decided to find out as much as you can about your disease, you are probably suffering from information overload by now. This is another point at which you need to remind yourself to breathe deeply, and to relax and meditate if you can, in order to get your mind to stop racing. What are you feeling right now? If you are feeling anxiety, close your eyes and slowly take 10 deep breaths.

If you don't live in an area where support groups are accessible, or you don't want to join a group, ask your doctor to recommend someone to talk to, someone who has had the disease. It doesn't matter how good the intentions of people who haven't had cancer are, they still don't really know how you feel. Only a fellow sufferer knows that.

Again, you may feel so overwhelmed with information that you feel as though you need more time to make your treatment decisions. It is perfectly all right in most circumstances to tell the doctors you want more time to think. After all, the tumor has probably been growing for several years, and waiting another few days before surgery won't make much difference. So if there is something important in your life you want to finish before surgery, I say go for it. However, if the surgeon has good reasons for not delaying, it's wise to listen. If you want a second opinion, ask for one; you are perfectly entitled.

In your case you may not have surgery to start with; radiation, chemotherapy, or hormone therapy may be recommended first, or instead of a surgical procedure. I will not attempt to go into the medical reasons for these alternatives here; I suggest you ask your oncologist and/or do your own research. Whatever your treatment, just find the relevant section in this journal and use it, and ignore the parts that don't apply to you.

What treatment has been recommended for you? What do you think about it?

THERE ARE MANY excellent books about the breast and breast cancer; probably the best and most detailed is *Dr. Susan Love's Breast Book*. Dr. Love, a surgeon, explains the various treatments in great detail and in accessible language. Other useful books are listed at the end of this journal.

A mastectomy is the procedure in which a whole breast is surgically removed. Partial mastectomy is another way of saying lumpectomy. In a lumpectomy just the tumor, and a small amount of tissue around it, is removed from the breast. While some women are glad that a partial mastectomy is recommended so that they won't have to lose the entire breast, other women want to have a mastectomy because they feel that the breast has betrayed them once already, and they don't want to give cancer another chance. Still others decide to have the other breast removed, as well, in order to lessen the chances of having cancer develop in that one. Lymph nodes under the arm are often removed during surgery for breast cancer and are then examined under a microscope to see if there are any cancer cells present there.

"It's easier to sell a lumpectomy than a mastectomy," Dr. J.T. Sandy says. I guess so. All I have to show for my surgery now is a discreet scar and a slight dent in the breast, along with a scar in my armpit where the lymph nodes were removed.

Some women would rather have a mastectomy. Elaine is one such woman: "My surgeon tried three times to convince me to have a lumpectomy. He said that in my case I fit the textbook picture for lumpectomy, and that with a tumor of less than two centimeters I didn't have to go through disfiguring surgery. I talked to friends in the radiography department where I work about my concerns about radiation therapy. Three of them are large-busted like I was, and they said they would have no hesitation about having a mastectomy given the large dose of radiation they would have to have if they didn't. The surgeon was concerned about the emotional aspect of mastectomy, but I said, 'The difference is that I have a choice, and I'm choosing mastectomy.' When I later found a thickening in the other breast, I told him I wanted a prophylactic mastectomy in that breast. When I got the pathology report on the other breast after surgery and they did find anomalies, it makes my decision look better all the time."

What are your feelings about the choice between a mastectomy or a lumpectomy?

STATISTICS: You probably had statistics about the possibility of recurrence and likelihood of survival quoted to you once they told you that your lump was malignant. If the cancer has spread to another part of your body (called metastasis) – for example if one or more of your lymph nodes tested positive for cancer – your chances of recurrence might sound quite stark when they are quoted in statistical terms. Mine certainly sounded stark to me: the oncologist told me I had a 66 percent chance of not having a recurrence if I had chemotherapy and radiation, which means that I had a 34 percent chance of having a recurrence even if I did. Put like that, the odds didn't sound good enough until I reminded myself of that old saw, the last refuge of the curmudgeon, about lies, damn lies, and statistics: the statistics they give you are a statement of mathematical probability, not a definite assertion that you will have a recurrence. I would like to be one of the 66 percent, and intend to be.

What were you told about your cancer?

Still having difficulty seeing myself as a cancer patient. Most of the time I can't believe it; other people seem more upset on my behalf than I am. There's a touch of not wanting to be identified with other people with cancer, too, if I'm honest. I don't want to be one of "them." This disease can come back at any time, anywhere, and kill you. I don't want it to. Doesn't that sound simple?

– from my own diary, April 1993

Caring, nurturing, that's what nurses do. That's not saying that physicians don't care, but they are scientists, too, and so they tend to get more focused on the statistics. It's changing, and they get a lot more psychosocial support training in medical school, but then they come out of med school and go into hospitals to be trained by people who are from the old school, and some of them rapidly lose their communication skill.

– Lenore Nicholson

DO YOU HAVE strong feelings about being someone who has been diagnosed with cancer? Have you ever thought how odd it is that we talk about someone being "diagnosed" with cancer? It is so indirect, impersonal. We don't say, "She got cancer," as if she owns it. It is almost as if it owns us and was just lying in wait to be discovered.

Very often it is the oncologists who give the medical facts to you, leaving the nurses to do a lot of the explaining and teaching. Nurses are usually aware of what the oncologists leave out, so they can fill in the gaps for you. Throughout my experience of cancer I found nurses, with all of their practical information, to be both a humanizing factor as well as extremely helpful.

On the following pages record your treatment options. When I was presented with some choices by my oncologist, I found it helpful to list advantages and disadvantages before I made my decisions. Making the list also identified areas about which I needed more information.

I wasn't convinced at first that I could accept having chemo. I read tons of information about it. I just wanted to know that it wasn't going to damage the healthy part of me.

– *Judy*

When I realized chemo
was an option, I did a
survey of my family doc-
tor, my surgeon, and a
friend who was a sur-
geon, and asked them:
"If this situation was
happening to your wife,
what would you do?"
They all said they'd rec-
ommend chemo. Having
that kind of support was
useful to me in making
my decision.

—Jo

Went to the clinic library
today. Wasn't sure what I
wanted, so the librarian
helpfully got me a video
and then showed me
where the files on alter-
native therapies were. All
the articles were critical,
of course, and not much
help except as a clue to
where Western medicine
is, or isn't, as I
discovered.

— from my own diary,
May 1993

Clearly the very hardest period was trying to choose a treatment. In addition to the anger I was often extremely upset, though too busy and frantic to have time to get depressed (I must have set a record for number of phone calls while trying to decide what to do). I had several days at first when I felt incredibly shaky, crying a lot, very agitated, close to falling apart, dwelling on fears of pain and thoughts of death . . . and then would come thoughts of all who are suffering on this planet at this moment, of all who have suffered in the past, and I would immediately feel a wave of peace and calm pass through me. I no longer felt alone, I no longer felt singled out; instead I felt an incredible connection with all these people, like we were part of the same huge family.

– *Treya Wilber,* Grace and Grit

AFRAID OF ITS long-term effects on the body, I was looking for alternatives to chemotherapy – any literature that could show with certainty that alternative or complementary therapies (as health care practitioners are now calling them) would give me a better chance than conventional medicine. Books told of various alternatives: some so far-out as to be beyond my ability to rationalize them, and some that made sense but didn't offer proof, just a vague sort of hope.

Anecdotal evidence wasn't enough; I needed something written in stone. I didn't know that such evidence did not exist anywhere and, to be cynical about it, will probably not exist until some drug company has figured out a way to make a buck out of it. Drug companies fund most of the research on new drugs, and although many drugs currently in use were developed from so-called folk remedies, the companies are generally not interested in anything that they cannot patent and market exclusively for themselves.

You will probably find that once you have made your decisions you will have more energy for day-to-day coping. Right or wrong, you have a course to follow, and a big stake in its outcome. Now is an excellent time to do meditations and visualizations. Use whatever comes naturally to you; it will calm you.

I have made my decisions. This treatment will give me my best chance of being well. May my body be strong and healthy.

Record your dreams here.

TREATMENT

Underlying much of the anguish that women experience as they move through diagnosis and treatment is a feeling of loss of control. There are two things that can help to alleviate this. The first is a shift in attitude from victim to participant. If you perceive surgery as a terrible thing that is being done to you against your will, you are a victim. On the other hand, if you are being offered a procedure that might very well save your life, and you choose it because you greatly value your life, you are a participant. That does not mean that you must look forward to the surgery. It simply puts you in a position of greater control because you have made the choice. The second way to gain control is to have a good rapport with your doctor. For me, having a surgeon who would respond to my questions and inspire my confidence was critical.

— Ronnie Kaye, *Spinning Straw into Gold*

What most women want
to know from me is: Is it
benign or malignant? If
it's malignant, what
does that mean?

– *Dr. J. T. Sandy*

CANCER IS A DRASTIC DISEASE and, unfortunately, the present treatments for it are almost equally as drastic. However, the knowledge that you are actively doing something to fight it and to help your body get better can give you the energy and impetus to get through it. Researchers are working on treatments that approach cancer from a different angle, so we can hope for less toxic treatment in the not-too-distant future. Meanwhile, we are stuck with what we have.

Because there are many different types of breast cancer and therefore many different forms of treatment, parts of this section of the journal may not apply to you. Just ignore those parts and go on to the next one.

SURGERY

IF YOU ARE NOT CLEAR about what the surgeon is planning to do, it is a good idea to get him or her to draw you a picture, or show you photographs, so you will know exactly what to expect. The risks of the surgery you are about to have should also be explained to you, as well as any possible side effects. You can then ask all the questions you want. If you are ready to take it in before surgery, you can also ask about exercises to do after the procedure, and whether physiotherapy after surgery is advisable. Some surgeons don't give you this information before surgery unless you ask; they feel, with some justification, that many patients don't hear a lot of what is being said if it isn't of immediate concern to them. If you don't think you need to know about exercise yet, make a note to ask later, and carry on with dealing with what you do need to know right now.

We have already mentioned surgery that involves removing lymph nodes from the armpit in order to see if any of the cancer cells have spread. This procedure – called axillary dissection – can have its own complications: ask your surgeon about them, particularly about the possibility of lymphedema (which is a swelling of the arm on the side that surgery has been done, caused by lymph fluid being unable to drain in the usual way). They usually take some extra tissue around the tumor to test whether the margins are "clear" of cancer. Again, you can ask your surgeon about this, or read about it. I wish I had asked more questions about axillary dissection at the beginning because the scar tissue has since caused me some discomfort, which might have been prevented.

Most women find one particular aspect of the surgery uncomfortable. After the axillary dissection is done, a drainage tube is usually inserted into your side for a few days. This can be exceedingly uncomfortable. Angie, for example, says: "When they pulled out those stupid drainage tubes, I thought, We send people to the moon, we can do microscopic eye surgery, surely somebody can figure out something better than sticking a large plastic tube into your skin, letting it heal over to the point where there's actually skin attached, and then yanking it out three days later. That really is prehistoric. I couldn't believe it. I understand that fluid collects, but can't they drain it out with a needle or something once a day? Can't they do something else? The pain was manageable, but it just seemed so stupid."

If you think you don't want to have a stream of people, loved ones, or not-so-loved ones coming to visit you in the hospital, try not to put the word out until you have been discharged. If that isn't practical, you can also tell the ward staff that you would like to restrict visitors. My wonderful friends, being who they are, visited a lot, and although coping with them made me tired, it also boosted my morale to see them. It is your choice. Another coping hint: If you haven't spent much time in the hospital, you may not know about hospital gowns, which open at the back and have a tendency to gape. Try to grab two gowns and wear one on top, open at the front. Thus dignity can be preserved.

How do you feel after surgery? Did you have a mastectomy or a lumpectomy? How do you feel emotionally? What can you do to make yourself feel better?

We have started to make terrible (and funny) cancer jokes. Started last night with thoughts of writing Harlequin Romances for people with cancer. Anyway, went to the surgeon, who removed the staples and about 110 ccs of fluid from my armpit; it's hardly surprising that I was stiff, sore and swollen. That was the good part. He also told me he had taken 18 lymph nodes and that one of them was "positive," which means that the cancer has spread and has the potential of spreading further, and that chemotherapy would probably be advised by the Cancer Agency. He also said one node out of 18 isn't bad, and that chemo "isn't as bad as it used to be." He said my tumor was "infiltrating ductal carcinoma

with poorly differentiated
cells," but that they
didn't yet know if it was
hormone-receptive, so I
won't know for a while
yet about whether I can
take tamoxifen instead of
having chemotherapy. So
there's no way out now.
It is the real thing. I'm
torn between anger and
crying. Damn it
all to hell.

– from my own diary,
April 1993

I walked every day. That became an obsession.
  – Judy

Treatment

73

I WALKED, TOO. I might only have made it halfway down the block some days, but at least I was outside. Even the dog was well behaved; she seemed to know something was wrong.

Have you had your pathology results? What were they?

What questions do you have? How do you feel about your body now?

After they did the biopsy and the hospital did the pathology, it looked like clean margins and that I'd just be having radiation, but when they checked the slides at the cancer clinic they said there were microscopic cancer cells, so then chemo got added in. I was not prepared for that. When they said yes it is cancer and you need surgery and radiation that was OK. It was exactly what I had planned out. I'd read Dr. Susan Love and things were going the way they were supposed to go. Chemo: no, no, no. It took a few hours to adjust to.

– Lynda

There was a period
where it was pretty hard
to look in the mirror,
because I'd had either
bandages or a very vivid
scar. One breast has a
big dent in it and a
scar. . . . I find the scar
really diminishing.
— *Angie*

ALL THE WOMEN I talked to emphasized the importance of doing what feels right for you. After all, you know your body better than anyone else. So if you want a mastectomy even though the surgeon says a lumpectomy is enough, go ahead and insist. It is your right. Get a second opinion if you want one. Trust your own instincts.

If you have had a mastectomy, you will be starting to come to terms with the loss of one, or both, of your breasts. This is a difficult time for many women; some cannot bring themselves to look at the scar. How will you handle it, or how did you handle it?

Funnily enough I can't say that when I had two breasts I was conscious of having breasts. I was definitely conscious when I had only one (with weight on one side and not the other). Now [after the second mastectomy] I feel absolutely the same as I did before all of this started if I'm not actually looking at my chest. With clothes on I have no concept walking around that I don't have breasts. It doesn't dawn on me.

– Elaine

YOU MAY FIND that you are mourning the loss of your breast or breasts. That is natural; they have been part of you for a long time and grief is an appropriate reaction. What are your thoughts?

It felt great to have a double mastectomy. I was offered a lumpectomy [before the second one] because the tumor was so small, but I said, "You must be joking," because I still had this scar area that was separate from the lump that I had been suspicious about the previous year and, in fact, when they did the pathology they found that there was an area of cancer in the region of the scar. You couldn't feel it, and it didn't show on the mammogram, but it was there.

– Brenda

I don't know if there's any real need to adjust to what it looks like to have a mastectomy. I looked at myself right away in the hospital. I was just lying there and I looked down to see what it looked like, and there was a big bandage on it, and it looked like a little bump, but nothing much. It's a shock. You don't ever expect it's going to look like that, that it's going to be so flat when they take the tissue out. Absolutely board-flat. As soon as I could get up I went into the bathroom and looked down to see what it looked like from the front, then from the side, and you sort of look like a 10-year-old on one side, kind of prepubescent, and then you turn to the other side and you've got this lump.

— Carol, diagnosed 1991

Chemotherapy

For the most violent diseases, the most violent remedies.
— Montaigne, *Essays, Book II*

IF YOU ARE READING this part of the journal, it probably means you are thinking about chemo or you have already made the decision to go ahead with it. We will not be going into the medical and scientific whys and wherefores of chemo, but we will talk about its effects, both on the emotions and on the body. Once you have made your decision to have chemotherapy, the most important thing is to try your mightiest to believe it will help you.

What are your feelings about chemotherapy right now? Anger, fear, acceptance? How do you feel about the prospect of losing your hair, if that is what is going to happen? If you are fearful or angry, pause and breathe deeply. Try to relax your neck and stomach muscles.

*I am fighting this disease
the best way I can.*

Twenty to 25 percent of patients have relatively few side effects. Some women keep working right through treatment. Ten to 15 percent have real difficulty. It's hard to get them to take four cycles of treatment. The rest have moderate side effects.

— *Dr. A. W. Tolcher*

I GUESS THOSE OF US who have to go through it would feel better if the doctors could tell us that chemo would cure us for sure, forever. No such luck: all we have to hang on to are those statistics that say we have a chance. The first thing to know is that not everybody has a bad time with chemo. It is safe to say that no one has fun, either, but there doesn't seem to be any way of telling ahead of time whether you will be one of the lucky ones who will "sail through it," as my surgeon put it.

The second most important thing to know is that treatment will come to an end eventually. There are some good books about it, and good videos have been made, as well. I suggest you ask your oncologist or nurse which ones are available in your area. In my own experience I found it particularly helpful to speak to women who had already had chemo. Again, what they had experienced was more real to me than anything the professionals could tell me.

SOME QUESTIONS TO ASK ABOUT CHEMOTHERAPY

- Why do I need it?

- How much will it improve my chances?

- Will I be an inpatient or an outpatient?

- How many treatments will I have, and over what period of time? How long will each treatment take?

- Which drugs will I be taking? Do I have a choice of drugs?

- What are the side effects of these drugs? How soon do they start? What can I do to reduce them?

- Will these drugs cause me to lose my hair? Will I lose all of my hair? Will it happen right away? Where is the best place to go for a wig? Are wigs expensive? Does health insurance cover wigs? Is any financial help available to obtain a wig?

- Will I lose weight? Will I gain weight? Will I have to change my diet? How long do the effects of chemotherapy last?

➤ Should I take time off from work?

➤ Will I need help at home?

Record your own questions about chemotherapy.

At the time I started to have chemo treatment you had it in the basement of St. Paul's Hospital with all the AIDS patients, in an incredibly depressing room, but you got used to it because the people were so wonderful. Then they moved into a ground-floor place, purpose-built in a new wing, where there was light, and that was much better.

– *Joan A*

CHEMO TREATMENT ROOMS have improved greatly. At the hospital where I was treated as an outpatient the waiting room was pleasant, the treatment rooms were nonthreatening, there was lots of light, and the people couldn't have been more helpful and supportive. Before leaving home each treatment day I made myself sit down, breathe deeply, and try to visualize how the drugs, the chemicals, were going to destroy the cancer cells still living inside me. I tried, with varying degrees of success, to visualize what the drugs were doing while they were in my body. Many of the visualizations for chemo suggested in support groups or in books are quite warlike and violent, and some women don't find them useful. Instead, you might like to visualize a stream of light searching out cancer cells and exposing them. There is, however, no right or wrong way to do visualizations, so find one that works best for you.

"Give yourself a goal for the end of treatment – a carrot," oncology social worker Elizabeth Dohan told me in the waiting room before my first treatment, suggesting that I give myself something to look forward to, a holiday perhaps. She was right. I gave myself permission to think about taking an unusual holiday after all of the treatment was finished. Thinking about it got me through many bad patches. If finances or your circumstances won't permit you to take an exotic holiday, dream about something you will be able to do. Write down your innermost goals.

The social worker showed me a picture of a cancer cell that looked big, weak, and confused, and that helped me to visualize using chemo to destroy these cells. I didn't buy into it completely and that worried me a little. I thought, I'll do the best I can with this, and that's OK, that's enough. I don't have to get perfect. What the chemo doesn't get rid of, I will get rid of through my own desire to live.

– Judy

I ALSO MADE the choice to continue going to work as much as I could. For about a week after each chemo treatment I stayed home, but I was able to work at least part-time. My employers lent me a modem so I could work on my computer at home, which I appreciated. Working gave me something to think about besides cancer. If you work outside the home, perhaps your employer would be willing to come to some similar arrangement. You may feel you just want to take the whole treatment period as sick leave: everyone's circumstances are different. Sometimes you may need to turn to your visualizations for extra help. Here are some other people's visualizations.

> *"When I was breast-feeding [before she was diagnosed], if the milk didn't come I would think of Niagara Falls. Then the milk would let down and I was able to feed my kid. So I thought if it worked for that, I could sit and visualize these humungous rivers running up my arm and hope a vein would pop up that the nurse could get the needle into."*
> – Debbie

> *"I have an image in my head of the chemo acting like Comet cleanser, going through my veins searching for cancer cells, scouring them out and leaving me all shiny inside. The image makes me smile."*
> – from my own diary, August 1993

> *"I visualized white cells growing, red cells growing, cancer cells being eaten up by the Pac-Man thing. I know that AIDS patients do that, and they can tell from the results of their bloodwork when they've been doing it and when they haven't. I didn't visualize the red cells one time, and they dropped off, so I realized I shouldn't forget to do it."*
> – Lynda

What are your own visualizations about chemotherapy?

I asked the social worker if she could give me the name of someone in the same boat as I was, and I talked to a woman who brought me some hideous socks that she wore during her chemo – she called them her "anti-nausea socks" – and said I wouldn't get sick if I wore them. So I wore them and didn't have much nausea. It was just in the background after the ondansetron [anti-nausea drug] was finished.

– *Judy*

As I mentioned earlier, everyone has a different reaction to chemotherapy: some people get very sick, others hardly at all. More effective antinausea drugs have appeared in the past few years, so most reactions are not as bad as they used to be.

Here are some random hints on how to cope with the effects of chemo. We will get to hair loss later on in this section.

- Nurses are usually a great source of practical information on coping with chemo.

- Ask your family and friends not to wear perfume or aftershave lotion around you. You may want to have unperfumed soap in the bathroom. Any strong odor can affect someone who is having chemo.

- Try to eat a light meal a couple of hours before having a treatment. It will give you strength.

- Don't eat your favorite foods if you are feeling sick. They will remind you later of chemo and you may not be able to eat them again.

Antinausea medication can make you constipated. I ate lentil soup and blueberries; Brenda ate prunes. Everyone is different. Just remember to keep drinking; fluids alleviate some of the problems associated with constipation. Dehydration can also contribute to fatigue.

It is all right if you can only eat a limited number of foods. What is important is that you are eating, so it doesn't matter if you keep eating the same thing. Eventually you will go back to a "normal" diet.

Lynda ate little but arrowroot cookies, while Judy ate sushi and Vietnamese salad rolls. When I could face them, I ate plain boiled eggs and black olives. You will notice that many foods taste different and that you often can't eat the things you really like. Some food textures may bother you. Don't worry. You will like them again when treatment is over.

If you are watching television, keep the remote control close to hand. I had no idea how many food commercials there are until I had chemo. If the antinausea medication doesn't work for you, insist on something else. It is usually possible to find some mix of medication that will help, but not always, unfortunately. Get the nurse to write the medication schedule down for you: it can seem awfully compli-cated if you have to work it out in the middle of the night when you are dozy and not feeling well.

If you get sores or a foul taste in your mouth, a solution of one tea-spoon of baking soda mixed into a glass of water and used as a rinse helps. Stay away from commercial mouthwashes that contain glyce-rin or alcohol; they will only dry out your mouth. Hard candy can sometimes help to get rid of the foul taste. Cranberry juice also works for many people.

Fresh air can help reduce nausea, too. Remove houseplants or cut flowers from your bedroom, or any of your other rooms, if the smell of the leaves, flowers, or potting soil bothers you.

Ask friends who want to help to go to the video rental store for you. Have them look in the comedy section. (*Fawlty Towers* saved my san-ity one night. *Mr. Bean* or Bernie Siegel's stand-up comedy routines might do the same for you.) Ask your friends to return the videos to the store afterward, if you don't feel up to it.

If possible, ask someone else to do the cooking on days when you are nauseated. Cooking smells can often trigger nausea. A good friend of mine made soup and froze it in little baggies so that I could defrost and heat it when I felt like it. Don't lie down right after eating; if you do, you will probably become nauseated.

Most people feel some fatigue during the treatment period. This is normal. Your sleep patterns may change.

You are more susceptible to infection during chemo, particularly seven to 10 days after each treatment, because the white cells that usually protect the body are reduced in number by the drugs. There is no need to panic, but do ask your doctor for details on what to do to avoid infection.

Remember: *you are not a failure if you have to vomit*. It has nothing whatsoever to do with willpower, and everything to do with the drugs inside you.

The following pages are blank so that you can draw pictures of what you think the chemotherapy drugs are doing to the cancer cells in your body. If you have trouble getting started, you may want to think of a vis-ualization you have used before and draw that. Perhaps you will dis-cover a hitherto unrecognized talent for drawing or painting.

I had given myself a year to deal with it [cancer] and then I thought it will be all over and I can get on with life, but then when I had chemo and got deathly ill that set me back. I was living by myself, and was sick in bed for two weeks after each chemo. Each one was so awful that I knew I had to be with people for three or four days afterward. Friends volun-teered to come and stay with me.

– *Lynda*

A friend brought cinnamon buns one chemo day and I haven't been able to face them since, and I love cinnamon buns. . . . Don't cook garlic! The first night of chemo, my husband was cooking Chinese food and it was game over. I'd felt wonderful up till then.
— *Debbie*

I cooked simple meals for the family, and I didn't eat very well myself – I ate crackers for a couple of days. My favorite drink was orange juice and soda water. The fizziness helped. I couldn't bear perfume and smoke, and I was very hyper and couldn't sit down. I felt I had to go for a walk after each treatment, before the rot set in. I had an incredible need for fresh air and exercise. Good physical exercise is important when you're doing chemo. It allows your body to flush out all the junk. I had heart arrhythmias, but by keeping fit I felt more regulated. Weight lifting and swimming may be too much, though.

– *Brenda*

THIS IS A really big deal for most of us, as you probably already know if you have been given the drugs that cause hair loss. The first thing to remember is that hair does grow back. Truly it does. My own came back much grayer (alas) but in tight little curls (it had been straight before), and I actually like it better now, although it has grown straighter with each haircut. I also lost most but not all of the other hair on my body, which I was much less well prepared for, such as my eyebrows, my eyelashes, my pubic hair, my underarm hair, and the hair on my legs.

We all have different reactions and experiences. In some way your hair defines you; it is one of the first things someone sees when they look at you. Some people undergoing chemo choose to get a wig, others wear decorative scarves or baseball caps, or they just go around bald. To be bald is fashionable right now; certainly in my neighborhood no one would look at you twice if you shaved your hair off. Here are some other people's observations on hair loss.

"I was told by the nurse that my hair would go two weeks after the first treatment. I was determined it wouldn't, but it did. One morning I had my hair. By afternoon it was coming out in big clumps. I sat on the beach and just let it go in the wind. I had a big hat and wore a scarf on my head at night. The hair came out quickly. I bought the most expensive wig I could find, then wore it one day to a movie and never again. I decided I could be comfortable without hair after watching that wonderful video about how to wear scarves. Scarves and neat earrings – I wanted to look like a gypsy, a little outrageous, in contrast to my conservative self. I liked a picture I saw of Sinead O'Connor bald."

– Judy

"I lost my hair on day 17 and hadn't combed my hair for two weeks prior to that. I thought that if I combed my hair it was really going to go. I looked at myself in the mirror, and thought, Oh, God, that's me. I'm sure that's the hardest part. My five-year-old insists on pulling my

wig off and showing everybody: 'Look, Mom's wearing a wig.' And I think, Shut your little mouth. I don't need this right now!"
– Debbie

"My reaction was 'Look, I'm molting.' It was devastating and I freaked out. I found a skullcap before I got the wig, and used scarves, and put a toque on at night. It took my hair six months to grow back. They don't tell you how long it takes to grow back in. It took my eyelashes and eyebrows longer to grow back."
– Val, diagnosed 1992

"I had already bought my wig and warned the hairdresser I'd be coming in for her to shave my head. I had decided I wasn't going to have hair falling out all over the place, I was going to be in control. I said, 'It's time.' She said, 'Are you sure?' I said, 'I'm sure.' So she shaved it off. She started at the back and did the front last, which was good. Thinking about it was worse than actually having it happen. It turns out I have quite a nice-shaped head, which I didn't expect. Then I put the wig on, the hairdresser styled it, and off I went. My head never got to being like a billiard ball, but pretty close. Chemo finished in September. I had about a quarter inch of hair by the middle of December. I was at a Christmas party and had to take the wig off because I was having a hot flash. They looked at my head and said, 'You've got lots of hair. You don't need to wear this anymore.' So I stopped wearing the wig. I hated it."
– Lynda

THERE ARE SOME ADVANTAGES to losing your hair, unlikely as that may seem. First, you don't have to buy shampoo. Second, if you usually shave your legs or underarms, you probably won't have to do that for a while. Third, you save money by not having to visit the hairdresser. Not all experiences of hair loss are negative.

"My hair came back the same boring old mouse color. The loss of the hair on my head was much less distressing than losing my eyebrows and eyelashes. I hadn't expected it and wasn't prepared for it. The

hair has never grown back under my right arm and is just wispy under the left arm. There are some compensations!"

– Joan A

The best of healers is
good cheer.

– *Pindar*, Nemean Odes

"I met a woman at the support group who made me laugh at the right moments, with plenty of black humor, and helped me let go."

– Judy

"I got upset about something during chemo and my friend said, 'Oh, Joan, do keep your hair on,' and we all howled with laughter."

– Joan A

HERE ARE SOME HINTS for coping with hair loss.

- Many women like to shave their heads when their hair starts to fall out so that they don't have to watch it come out in clumps. Others get their hair cut really short before treatment starts.

- Use a gentle shampoo.

- If your head gets cold, wear a soft cap. Hair is great insulation; without it you may find your head gets especially cold at night.

- There are videos about scarf tying if you decide to go that route. Check your local library or breast cancer center for more information.

- Many people recommend that you buy your wig before treatment begins.

I bought a wig before my treatment began, but because my face lost color during chemo, the wig turned out to be too dark. Also, the low-growing hair on the back of my neck didn't fall out completely and showed at the point where the wig ended if I forgot to shave it. Make sure your wig fits you well. Ask your nurse, social worker, or cancer society for the name of a good wig supplier.

As YOU START to lose your hair, you may find it useful to be in a support group. I was terrified about what was happening to my mind and body during chemo, and was immensely relieved when I discovered that it was also happening to most of the other women I talked to. It is a dark subject, and we all had tears to cry, but we usually found much to laugh about, as well.

On the blank pages that follow write about your own chemo experience: how it affects you, how your body feels, and especially how it affects your mind. Somebody I met while I was going through chemo told me about "CRS Syndrome." CRS stands for "Can't Remember Shit," which seems to sum up nicely what has happened to me and my mind, since I can no longer remember who it was who told me about it. Other people talk about "chemo brain," and women who are catapulted into menopause by chemo often wonder whether what is happening to their emotions is caused by treatment or the actual onset of menopause. (We will talk about treatment-induced menopause later.) It could be that the chemo drugs and the antinausea medication themselves affect the brain somehow.

I thought I was getting Alzheimer's. Talk about not remembering things. At work I would get numbers transposed, and I thought it was just me, though I hadn't had problems like that before. I still get them mixed up! I forget names, too. I'm afraid to use them in case I get it wrong. Menopause and chemo were all intermingled. It's a wonder I knew who I was.

– *Val*

YOU MAY FIND it helpful to include your antinausea medication schedule here. I could never have remembered how often to take each different pill if I hadn't written it down. Allow yourself to feel terrible, if that is in fact how you feel. Remember that you will feel better later on.

By accepting these chemotherapy drugs, I am inviting them to seek out the cancer cells, to destroy them, and to make me well.

YOUR EMOTIONS will probably be all over the place while you are going through treatment. Behaving normally is not an option for most of us. My own experience was to have feelings of sadness and otherworldliness during and after chemo treatments. Everyone has different reactions.

"I was angry during chemo. I beat the shit out of my bed with an aluminum baseball bat. A psychologist friend living down the street recommended it, and I felt much better afterward."
  – Judy

"I get angry more often, which is probably justified all the time! Maybe I'll become more outspoken. You can say anything you want. It doesn't bloody well matter once you've had a diagnosis of cancer. You can say what you think. Little things do bug me more. Maybe I'm just more aware of it."
  – Debbie

"I couldn't sleep and got claustrophobic. I couldn't draw the curtains. I didn't like the dark. I was very hyper and couldn't sit down. . . . They should remember that there's all sorts of other baggage going on in people's lives [as well as cancer]. I was a basket case because my elder daughter was just about to have a biopsy for suspected Hodgkin's disease and I was worried about her."
  – Brenda

"It's hard to say if I had mood swings, because I found during treatment time that all my friends protected me against having to deal with the real world, so I never really got tested. It was an incredibly stress-free time. I could see how people who got sick could decide they'd like to stay sick because it's a safer environment to be in. . . . I'd have a little cry every once in a while, but I felt fairly even-keeled, even through chemo. I lost my sense of humor through chemo, though."
  – Lynda

How are you coping?

THE PERIOD WHILE I was undergoing chemotherapy was one time in my life that I was really glad to be living alone. I was happy to see my friends at times of my own choosing, or to talk to them on the phone, but I don't know how I would have handled it if someone else had been around all the time. An answering machine is a must. I felt disgusted with my own body. There I was with no hair, vomiting or feeling like vomiting most of the time, not comfortable lying down or sitting down or standing up, with my mind somewhere out in space. Yuck. But not everyone feels the way I did.

> *"Every chemo treatment was just awful, so I knew I had to stay with people after each one for three or four days. Then I needed to come home because I wanted to sleep in my own bed."*
> – Lynda

> *"The things I needed – scarves, the wig – my partner was part of that. After chemo we'd go wandering through stores and he'd buy me something sometimes. After the first chemo, I decided I needed a juicer and would only eat organic food. I would drag him to the health food store, and he hates shopping. He was angry and so was I. I was feeling like I was on the other side of the world, as if there was a glass case around me, not part of the world outside. I felt disconnected from other people. I remember sitting in the garage with him one day, and I said, 'I'm so angry I could smash everything in sight.' He just sat with me and listened, which was exactly what I needed. I vented, I felt better, he was there for me. He won a lot of points and did exactly what he should, though he was probably terrified. It's all about expressing anger in front of another person. It made me able to relate to his anger, which had always scared me. It gave me permission to be angry. I let off steam and then I got connected to him again."*
> – Judy

"I think I was quite lucky. I had antinausea pills. I didn't feel in control of myself really, but if I went to bed as soon as possible for a couple of hours after each treatment, then I felt all right again, quite normal and able to cope."

– Joan A

Do you prefer to be by yourself if possible after a treatment, or would you rather have company? How do you feel during and after a treatment?

IT CAN BE HARD to sort out everything that happens to your body while you are going through chemo. I felt cold and disoriented for a few days after each treatment, but I also experienced hot flashes, mood swings – the whole lot – and I didn't know whether to attribute these symptoms to menopause or to chemo. Ask your oncologist if there is anything you can do to counter these side effects. If your periods stop, they may come back after six months or even a year.

Your mind is just as important as your body. How do you really feel right now?

Seventy percent of women go through loss of periods. Fifty percent of those get it back afterward. It has to do with their age. In younger women there is usually no change. You are likely to lose your periods if you are older. There is no way to protect the ovaries. There is some evidence that women who go through menopause at chemotherapy do better, so it is not necessarily a curse that you lose your periods. It may be a blessing.

– Dr. A. W. Tolcher

I thought I had gone into menopause. My period stopped in August. I was having hot flashes and night sweats, and my GP told me that was it. I asked if I should give away my tampons, and she said yes. Then in April it started again, but not regularly. It comes and goes. No wonder you're losing your mind. There's too much assault on the old body.

– *Lynda*

A nice thing happened today: a card from Jo, congratulating me on having come through chemo. It made me feel wonderful; only someone who's been through it can appreciate what an ordeal it truly is.
— from my own diary, August 1993

BECAUSE CHEMOTHERAPY is such an ordeal for most of us, congratulations are definitely in order at the end of treatment. What a marvelous feeling it was not to have to go back for any more chemo! Sick as I felt, knowing that did wonders for my morale. Another friend sent me a beautiful bunch of flowers to mark the occasion, and even though I had to put them outside because my sinuses were acting up at the time, looking at them gave me tremendous pleasure.

After my last treatment I remember saying to the chemo nurses (who were a wonderful bunch) that, although I meant no offense, I hoped I never had to see them again.

How are you feeling?

Did anyone in particular help you while you were having treatments? Perhaps you would like to note the details here so that you can do something about it later. Did anyone (or anything) make you particularly angry or sad? What did they do or not do?

It's so nice to have it over with. I found I was really dreading each treatment, anticipating it all week long.

– Debbie

FOR SOME WOMEN hair starts to grow back before chemo is over; other women don't see anything for a month or two. Different people have different reactions.

> *"At the clinic I asked the young doctor if he thought my hair could grow back through the thick skin that seems to have appeared on my head. I don't think he was an expert on hair, but I whipped off my wig and he peered at my scalp and said he couldn't see anything wrong. Later on I inspected it closely and think some hair is growing in in places. My scalp looks as if it's been dyed by the wig, but I guess it's hair coming through, after all."*
> – from my own diary, September 1993

> *"I kept watching for my hair to come back in, and when it did, I felt very tender toward it. I really liked it. It was a wonderful, miraculous thing to see this almost baby hair, like a chicken's down coming back on your head. I liked to touch it because it felt so nice. For a long time I wouldn't have it cut because I thought it was too precious."*
> – Joan A

If you lost your hair, has it started to come back in yet? How does that feel? How did you feel when you first saw it or felt it coming back in? What are you going to do with your wig, if you have one?

Chemotherapy is over. Now I can concentrate on getting well again.

What would you most like to do with the rest of your life? If you could have the choice of anything in the world, what thing would you most like to do today? If that is not realistic right now, what can you do today to celebrate?

Record your dreams here.

HORMONE THERAPY refers to a number of different treatments designed to reduce the level of female hormones in the body. Estrogen, which is one of the female hormones, is believed to contribute to the growth of some breast tumors. If your oncologist thinks you are a likely candidate for hormone therapy, he or she is the best one to answer your questions about it. In short, hormone therapy can mean taking drugs, or having the ovaries removed surgically or by radiation.

We will talk about tamoxifen here, the most common drug used to reduce or block the body's production of estrogen. Whether or not your oncologist will recommend tamoxifen for you depends on many factors, the main one being your menopausal status: it is most effective in postmenopausal women whose tumors are estrogen-receptor positive. Long words, but your oncologist will probably have explained all of this to you. Most books about breast cancer have sections on tamoxifen and other hormone therapies. It is worth the effort to find out about such treatments before talking to your doctor.

At the time of writing, studies are being done on a drug called Taxol. Taxol has been used to combat ovarian cancer, but it is also being tested on breast cancer patients and appears to have a high response rate. Some oncologists believe it may turn out to be of more use than tamoxifen, but the results of the studies won't be in for another two to three years yet.

You may want to ask your oncologist about tamoxifen. Here are some suggested questions.

- Why are you recommending it for me?

- What will it do?

- Will taking it after the completion of chemotherapy increase my chances of staying well?

- What are the risks of taking it?

- What side effects can I expect? Short-term? Long-term? How can I monitor these? Can I reduce them by splitting the dose?

- For how long will I have to take it?
- What form does the drug take?
- Will I have to pay for it?
- Can I use oral contraceptives while I am taking it?
- Should I become pregnant while taking it?

List your own questions.

WOMEN I HAVE SPOKEN TO talk about the menopause-like side effects they have experienced while taking tamoxifen. Brenda, for example, says: "I'm on tamoxifen. They say my hot flashes and night sweats are related to it." Other women have mentioned cold spells, mood swings, weight gain, depression, nausea, dry skin, problems with their eyes, or unusual vaginal discharge. I emphasize, though, that each woman is different: you may not experience any of these side effects. This is another time when a support group could provide information that will help you to make a decision. If hormone therapy has been recommended for you, how do you feel about it? List the advantages and disadvantages as you see them.

Record your dreams here.

YOUR RADIATION ONCOLOGIST can explain how radiotherapy is used to fight cancer, and why it is being recommended for you. In many ways radiation is easier to visualize and to understand than chemotherapy. One advantage is that it is relatively painless, unless you develop a burn (as a few women do). Another advantage is that you don't lose your hair if they are not aiming the rays at your head. What the technologists are doing each time is pointing high-energy rays at a specific part of your body for a short time in order to kill cancer cells. If you have had a lumpectomy, you are probably being given radiation to get rid of any cancer cells that may still be lurking in that breast.

How do you feel about radiation therapy? What have you been told about it? What have you read? What are you concerned about specifically? What questions would you like to ask the oncologist? Here are some sample questions.

- How many treatments will I have, and how long will they take?

- Does it hurt?

- Will they be radiating my armpit?

- Will they have to radiate any of my organs?

- If my left side is being radiated, will it damage my heart?

- How often during the treatment period will I see the radiation oncologist?

- What are the possible side effects? What should I do if I have them?

- Will I be fatigued?

- What will my breast look like afterward? Will there be much change?

- Are there any long-term effects?

Write your own questions here.

The clinic called: radiation starts Monday. At the thought of more treatment I went into fear mode again and almost got nauseated. I want to cry a lot, too. I wanted to read, but couldn't because my mind was racing. I wish I weren't so weary.

– from my own diary, August 1993

RADIATION MAY BE easier to cope with than chemo, but it has its own side effects and requires a similar commitment from you. It requires a time commitment, as well. I had to go in for radiation treatment every day, except for weekends, for 16 days. I found the daily trek to be tiresome and enervating. Radiation therapy is also essentially a technical process, and many women find it somewhat dehumanizing. The technologists are very busy, and don't usually have much time for social niceties, so be prepared for that. What follows are some experiences others have had with radiation treatment.

> *"I went to the clinic to be measured for radiation today. They painted lines on my chest to show the boundaries of the radiation area, and made some tiny, permanent tattoo marks. They make these marks so they will always be able to tell where you've had radiation before because they can't radiate the same area twice. I found there were too many people staring at me in that tiny examination room. They had asked me if it was okay for all the people to stay (two were students, I believe), and I could have told them to go away, but I didn't. The actual treatments took about one minute each, one for each side of my breast. You go into an unfriendly sort of room, full of this huge machine [a linear accelerator], and the technicians spend a lot of time positioning you on a movable bed with your arm above your head. Then they tell you not to move, and leave the room while the machine whirrs at you. I tried not to panic, and found it helped if I counted how many seconds each dose lasted. I have to go once a day for three weeks and a day, except for weekends."*
> – from my own diary, August 1993

> *"It didn't make me particularly tired and I had no skin problems. I virtually sailed through it and didn't give it much thought. It was icing on the cake after the chemo."*
> – Judy

"I don't know if the lymphedema was enhanced, but as far as my skin was concerned, I got a touch of heat rash at the end. I put cortisone cream on it. I got more tired afterward, but I was tired, anyway, with menopause and chemo, et cetera."
   – Lynda

"I didn't have much problem while having it. My husband had gone on ahead to England without me. I had the children at home, so I could go to bed early without being antisocial. I had horrible flaky skin, and I thought, At least I'm the only person who has to look at this. After about a week in England, I seemed to become very weak for a while. It upset me greatly that I couldn't cut the grass in one go, and it was a couple of months before I felt normal again."
   – Joan A

"I had 16 doses of radiation and got a burn after I finished. It accumulates. My breast was sore from it, but isn't anymore, though I often have pains in that breast. It'll ache. It's not sharp pains."
   – Angie

AS I SAID EARLIER, I found it quite a trial to have to make the journey every day to receive radiation therapy; it was a daily reminder that I had cancer and that treatment was not over yet. Just after radiation finished I had to go on a business trip, and I felt the most astonishingly sharp pains in the radiated breast as the airplane descended to the runway. I guess the change of pressure was causing the pain, but I certainly wasn't prepared for it. I have done quite a lot of flying since and haven't felt the pains again.

It is possible that you will have the odd sharp pain in your breast that has nothing to do with cancer. During surgery some nerve damage may occur and the pain you feel later is often the nerves trying to come back to life.

Everyone has a different reaction to radiation. Yours will probably be different, too. What is your treatment schedule? How do you feel about it?

Visualize, as you are receiving the treatment, that the machine is beaming a clean, pure light to that area of your body, targeting the bad cells and making room for the good cells to take over again.

List some visualizations for radiation therapy that work for you. It might help to start out by drawing a picture of yourself and the radiation. Make the picture warlike or peaceful. It is up to you.

I am taking all the steps I can to become healthy again.

How do you feel about the radiation treatment itself now that it has started? If there is anything happening that you aren't comfortable with, you are perfectly entitled to say so. Better out than in, as the old cliché goes. Rehearse here, if you like.

Are there any side effects you need to tell the oncologist about, or
questions you need to ask?

HERE ARE SOME HINTS on how to cope with radiation:

- Don't wear light-colored clothing when you go in for the planning session. The ink from the lines they draw on you may rub off onto your clothes.

- Try to wear a two-piece outfit each time you go so that you will only have to take your top off when they treat you.

- Because you won't be able to use creams or deodorants that contain aluminum or other metals, cornstarch can be used as a substitute.

- Some women are more comfortable not wearing a bra, others find that an old, loose bra gives them the best support. At any rate, you probably won't want to wear a tight bra, or one that has an underwire.

Your experience may be different, but I had unusually vivid dreams during my radiation therapy. Perhaps it was the fact that there was a large machine directing *Star Wars*-type rays at me every day that caused my imagination to take wing. On the following pages record any dreams you have had during radiation treatment.

Now we will assume that your radiation therapy has ended. Whatever your experience was, we can hope the treatment did what it was supposed to do. Congratulations – you came through it! Another milestone passed on the way back to better health.

How do you feel about being at the end of these treatments?

IF YOU HAVE come to the end of your treatment altogether, you may feel like celebrating. On the other hand, you may be feeling too tired. Still, try to do something nice for yourself at this time, even if you don't have the energy to go out on the town. Perhaps just being able to sit in a chair quietly by yourself is all the celebrating you need to do.

Some women feel anxious when their treatment period comes to an end. Up until now you have been actively working with the treatments – doing something to further your recovery. Without that you may experience a letdown: you are out on your own and you have time to think about the future. If this is how you are feeling, there is a section toward the end of this book called "Where Do I Go from Here?" that you may find useful.

You may feel that while your friends and family were attentive and helpful during treatment, they are now beginning to forget that you were "ill." This could be a good time for you to get into a support group. There is nothing like talking to a bunch of people who have been through a similar experience. I found being in the group removed much of my immediate fear; it was immensely reassuring to meet women still alive and well many years after their diagnosis. If groups aren't your thing, there are several books about coping with chronic illnesses and the uncertainty they bring, or you might consider counseling. Ask your doctor what help is available if you feel you need it. Just remember that what you have been through is traumatic, to say the least, and that you will probably need time to recover. Go easy on yourself.

Record the dreams you have after your radiation therapy is completed.

It must be acknowledged . . . that much healing occurs outside the realm of science.

– *Ivo Olivotto, Karen Gelmon, and Urve Kuusk,* Breast Cancer: All You Need to Know to Take an Active Part in Your Treatment

WHATEVER YOU CALL IT – some people refer to it as "complementary," others as "alternative," medicine – a lot of people with cancer use one form of complementary therapy or another, either along with conventional medicine or by itself. Why do we use alternatives? Mainly because conventional Western medicine cannot offer a surefire cure for breast cancer.

Using complementary therapies can give you a sense of being in control of at least part of your getting-well program. It also enables you to take care of that other part of your body, the larger part, that is healthy and normal. In my own case, I found that using other therapies gave me a sense of hope for the future, which I was unable to extract from the dry medical statistics oncologists use. It also helped me to believe that I was taking a leading role in making myself well again.

What are your thoughts on complementary therapies?

I always have trouble with these words that the medical profession comes up with for the nonscientific therapies. Their other favorite word is *unproven*. I think they should be called something like *supportive therapies,* or *health-enhancing therapies.* Let's make a new word that relates to how we the users view these therapies.

– Judy

Alternative medicine is a
part of healing. It
empowers you in a way
that chemo doesn't.
Being a "patient" means
"sit and wait." Medicine
should be about your
having a choice. Shop
around, and don't
expect miracles.
— *Silvia Wilson*

YOU SHOULDN'T LEAVE your usual skeptical consumer skill at the door when you are considering complementary medicine. Caveat emptor – let the buyer beware – applies here, too. Although claims made for some therapies can be absurd, some do have value. Do your research. Admittedly research can be hard to come by, since very little scientific testing has been done on these therapies. I am glad to say that at the time of writing some testing on complementary medicine is being done, mainly at the instigation of women living with breast cancer, and we can hope for results that will convince skeptical medical professionals of its value. However, some excellent books have been published recently (you will find a list of suggested titles at the end of this journal) that might help you to make a decision about which therapies to explore or use. You can also talk to other women with breast cancer to find out what they are doing.

Visualization, meditation, therapeutic touch, and yoga all fall under the heading of complementary therapy. They can certainly reduce stress and, in some cases, can also reduce pain and the side effects of treatment. Most of the women I talked to for this book told me they had used some form of visualization and that their experience had been positive.

My own choice was to see a naturopath and a doctor of traditional Chinese medicine as well as the cancer doctors throughout the treatment period and afterward. I decided to take Chinese herbs because the way traditional Chinese medicine works (by looking at the whole body, not just the parts in question) made sense to me. I also had acupuncture treatments during chemo and afterward, took antioxidants and extra vitamins, meditated, used visualization with and without audiotapes, changed my diet, and gave up caffeine. I wanted to give my body the best possible chance of getting well again, and these things seemed right for me.

I also made a point of telling my oncologist about my extracurricular therapies, in case anything I was doing interfered with my chemo or radiation treatments. Oncologists tend not to know much about complementary medicine, although some have been known to refer patients to naturopaths and other practitioners. The B.C. Cancer Agency, my local cancer hospital, is enlightened enough to run excellent relaxation programs and support groups. I consider myself fortunate to have been able to participate in them.

Don't feel that you have to do any of these things if they don't feel right for you. The choice is entirely up to you. There are many different alternatives, as the following comments demonstrate.

"Alternative medicine is getting more recognition. Physicians sometimes suggest patients should try other things. Twenty or 30 years ago immunology was considered 'quack' medicine, now it's leading-edge. Neuropsychoimmunology was considered crackpot five years ago, now it's being seriously researched. People are hearing about it from friends. Medicine doesn't have all the answers. The patients that want to take charge are the ones who come [to see me]."

– Dr. Lawrence Chan, D.C., N.D., naturopathic physician

"I used visualization, a lot of therapeutic touch, massage. I do relaxation stuff every night, and have done right from the time I had surgery. I'd visualize peace and harmony flowing into my body, and stress and disease being wiped out. I tried to do a visualization of getting rid of lymphedema, but couldn't get a handle on that so I quit. Since my second cellulitis [infection of the soft tissue], I've also been getting acupuncture. I do tai chi and the sun salutation every day. I've started meditating, too."

– Lynda

"I started reading, and bought several books for reference. I read Austin and Hitchcock's Breast Cancer: What You Should Know (but May Not Be Told) About Prevention, Diagnosis and Treatment. *I thought she [Cathy Hitchcock] was very brave for not having gone with any of the conventional therapies. I certainly wouldn't be able to do that. It's too scary. I'd rather go with the known treatments."*

– Debbie

"I took up tai chi. It makes sense, you get the exercise, but it's not strenuous. Meditation and yoga aren't my bag, and I wouldn't be able to devote myself to it, but tai chi is just plain good exercise and good for stress reduction. I'm not an aerobics person."

– Elaine

It is reasonable to expect the doctor to recognize that science may not have all the answers to problems of health and healing. But it is not reasonable to expect him to give up the scientific method in treating his patients.

– *Norman Cousins,*
Anatomy of an Illness

If we had effective
therapies, these things
would disappear. Most
people have a burning
desire to live.
– *Dr. A.W. Tolcher*

WHILE I WAS UNDERGOING treatment, several people mentioned that they were praying for me. Although I am not religious, I found it comforting to know that prayers were being said for me, and I have recently read newspaper reports of a study in which it was shown that patients who were prayed for during an illness actually did better than other patients. By the time this book is published, someone will probably have disproven that study, but it is a good thought nevertheless, and I have never heard of anyone actually being harmed by prayer. We should not underestimate its power.

A number of women mentioned that therapeutic touch had helped them. It is usually the nurses who know about these kinds of complementary therapies, so if therapeutic touch interests you, ask one of them if they know who can help you.

Record your dreams here.

I have lousy veins, so getting an IV started was a major production every time, so a friend made me a specific relaxation tape for my chemo. Then I'd get therapeutic touch to make everything go as smoothly as possible. It worked.

– *Lynda*

I will be able to look back and know that I have done everything I can to help my body get well again.

A Safe Place
136

RECONSTRUCTION OR NOT?

*I didn't try reconstruction immediately – it was suggested
I wait a year – and I wanted to do it because implant surgery was
cheaper than a prosthesis, and because I'm a swimmer and wearing a
prosthesis is a drag. I tried the saline implants twice, but it seemed clear
that my body didn't want them, and it felt great when they were finally
taken out. I have bathing suits made for me now.*

– Jo

It is a question we ask ourselves – what's it going to be like being one-breasted in a two-breasted world, or a double-breasted world as we called it then? I suddenly realized one day that I was looking at all the women walking toward me and staring right at their breasts, realizing that in a week's time I wasn't going to look like that, that I'd be lopsided, and I wasn't very happy at the prospect. At the same time I wasn't happy at the prospect of having cancer cells in my body that could kill me, and if losing the breast was going to keep me alive, then I was willing to make that bargain. I had reconstruction for purely cosmetic reasons. The decision took a long time to make, and I changed my mind several times,

IF YOU HAVE had a mastectomy, you may have to make a decision whether to have the missing breast reconstructed, whether to use a prosthesis, or whether to do nothing at all. Perhaps you have decided to have a prophylactic mastectomy on the other side, as well. If you have had a lumpectomy, this chapter is probably not for you, unless you have had a large amount of tissue removed. Your cancer surgeon can refer you to a plastic surgeon, who will tell you what your options are. Reconstruction may depend on how much tissue is left after your cancer surgery, along with other factors, but each case is evaluated on its own.

There are different types of breast reconstruction to consider. Talk to your surgeon. Talk to women who have had mastectomies; the cancer societies have programs that put women with breast cancer together to share their experiences one-on-one. Support groups can also put you in touch with the information you need.

Remember that although the decision whether to have reconstruction can be made before your mastectomy, and some surgeons will strongly recommend that you decide prior to the procedure, you don't have to make a choice at this point if you are not quite sure it is what you want. The diagnosis of cancer and mastectomy itself can be hard enough to deal with without also having to make a decision about whether to have reconstruction right away. Some women choose to have reconstructive surgery years after their mastectomy.

The important thing is to get all the information you need before you make your decision. It is your decision, no one else's, so *you* have to be comfortable with it.

Single women may have different reactions from women who have partners. For example, a single woman may be anxious about how a new lover will perceive her body; women with longtime partners may be less concerned about what other people think. Some women may fear that they will lose their sexuality when they lose a breast. Again, a support group can help, and so can counseling.

Here are some questions to ask the surgeon.

- What kinds of breast reconstruction have you done? How many have you done?

- What type do you recommend for me? Why? How many times will you have to operate?

- Should I have it done immediately, or can it wait till I am ready?

- Will the new breast look any different from the other one? If it is going to look very different, should I have the other one changed at the same time so they will match?

- Can you show me pictures of how women look after having the type of reconstruction you are recommending for me? I would like to see good and bad results in order to understand what can happen.

- What will the reconstruction look like as I get older?

- Is reconstruction major surgery? How will I feel afterward?

- Is lymphedema more likely to occur?

- How soon after surgery will I be able to go back to work? Will the surgery affect the work I do inside or outside my home?

- Will reconstructive surgery interfere with other treatments?

- Will it interfere with detecting another cancer later on?

List your own questions here.

but I went to the support group one day and a woman there had just been to pick up her new [fake] nipple at the clinic. She was delirious with happiness and pulled up her sweater to show us what she looked like, and I was knocked out. I thought that if it was going to look so natural, then I'd have it done, too. I'm glad I did.

– Carol

List the advantages and disadvantages of reconstruction as you see them.

How do you see yourself? Try doing a self-portrait of before and after surgery, with and without reconstruction.

ELAINE'S DECISION to have a mastectomy was based on having undergone four biopsies in one year that showed atypical cells. Her surgeon was concerned about the emotional aspects of the surgery, but she told him, "The difference is that I have a choice, and I am choosing mastectomy." She also didn't want to have radiation. Later she had biopsies done on the other breast, which showed more atypical cells, so she decided to have a prophylactic mastectomy done on that side, as well. After the surgery they found more anomalies; she feels she made the right decision: "I didn't make the decision lightly. There's a certain amount of erotic and sexual pleasure that I gain from my breasts and my sense of sexuality. Funnily enough, I feel less awkward now than I did then. I was a 38D, and if I didn't wear the prosthesis [after the first mastectomy], I felt very lopsided. One day I was up at the mall with a friend – it was warm and I'd left my jacket in the car and all I was wearing was a golf shirt – and my friend said, 'What's that guy staring at?' I said, 'Oh, probably me,' because I wasn't wearing the prosthesis on that side."

Here are what three other women who have dealt with the question of reconstruction say:

"I really didn't mind the surgery, the double mastectomy. I looked forward to it. In fact, I couldn't wait to get it done. And in terms of the prosthesis, it gives you more flexibility. I can decide to be a size 2 or a size 9. I can be voluptuous in the evening and have a little prosthesis at other times. I wear them just about all the time. The only time I didn't was in the summer when it was really hot and I was doing housework. I still feel like the same person. Being alive and able to get back doing things outweighed the importance of having body parts missing – it was not important."
– Brenda

"The surgeon put in a few CCs of saline when he put the expander in [at the start of reconstruction], and it was like going through puberty again – there was the little bump where there had been nothing before. People ask if the surgery hurt, but it didn't. There was nothing left there to hurt. I've talked to women who have had

pain, and I think it's their muscle that hurts because it's been
pushed and pulled."
    – Carol

"I had a radical mastectomy in 1971. There was very little discomfort afterward, and I have no scars. They did a skin graft, and I had two or three weeks of radiation, but no reconstruction. If anyone ever questions my decision, I just say, 'Well, I'm the one that's still walking around.' It makes no difference to one's intimacy, though it did take a while to heal. I've never regretted the decision."
    – Adine

How are you feeling right now? Have you made your decision? Do you feel better for having made it? If you are still undecided, write it out.

Record your dreams here.

TAKING CARE OF YOUR MIND

I came out of the abyss when I realized suddenly that although all this stuff was happening to me, I felt well and was active and alive. I felt I could manage it all and be alive if I just lived one day at a time.

– Judy

It took me a long time to cry. I went to the relaxation class six months after surgery. The lights were down and the music started, and I was lying on a mat. They were talking about relaxing your toes and your hair follicles and all the rest of it, and the tears started running down my face. Oh, I was so embarrassed. I let go because I felt safe in that room. I felt it was all right after that to cry in the quiet of the shower, and I did. I had thought that it was probably not very good for my prognosis to be crying, that you have to pick yourself up, dust yourself off, and keep on going, but crying does help.

– *Carol*

THE CARE AND FEEDING of your mind is every bit as important as the treatment you are taking for your body. Previously I discussed some techniques for relieving fear, anger, and grief – relaxation, visualization, meditation, exercise, taking part in support groups, talking to a counselor. All the feelings you are having are entirely justified: cancer is a fearsome disease. Once we have been diagnosed with it we have to deal with the consequences, whether we want to or not. It is okay to let go.

As I have already mentioned, crying is good therapy. And just about every woman I have talked to told me that she got through her experience of cancer by taking it one day at a time. My own choice was to see a psychologist, starting while I was having chemo, because I was being overwhelmed by my emotions and didn't want to dump all over my friends. Other women handle things quite competently and calmly on their own. There is no right way to deal with the diagnosis or treatment of cancer.

Everybody has a different mechanism for keeping their sanity. How are you doing it? Are there particular people helping you by being there when you need them, or are you coping by yourself?

You may remember that in "After the Diagnosis" I talked briefly about setting aside the fear of immediate death. What we have to do is acknowledge the fear, then start facing the fact that although it probably isn't going to happen today, right this minute, we are going to die someday. We all are. Life always ends in death.

Our feelings about death are vastly more complicated than that, of course. None of us wants to die slowly and painfully, and we like to think that what we do and who we are will live on after us. If we had our way, we would live out our full term in good health and happiness, dying surrounded by those who love us, at the end of a life in which we had achieved everything we ever wanted. This might happen to characters in novels and old Hollywood movies, but seldom to real mortals.

We can't spend the rest of our lives worrying about the inevitable. What we have to do is come to terms with the idea of not being here forever, then get on with making the rest of life as good as we can. Sounds easy, doesn't it? To share my own experience with you, it has only been recently – four years after diagnosis – that I think I have come to terms even a little bit with my own mortality.

Think about it: history is populated by dead people. They lived, and then they died. Everybody died eventually. I am not sure why I find that a comforting thought, but I do. What we do with our lives does live on after we have gone; we can see that around us every day. No matter how much time we have left we can still make life happier for ourselves now. It is a goal: how you do it doesn't matter.

If you feel like recording your thoughts about death and dying, jot them down here.

It's made death a lot less frightening. It's awful not to be here, but death's not so mysterious, I guess. When you face life-threatening illness it just doesn't become such a big deal. It's not that I don't want to live. It's just that I don't think dying is such a big deal. You're either going to die now or you're going to die later. Almost everyone dies of either heart disease or cancer if they live to be old enough.

– *Carol*

When my father was
dying of liver cancer, I
wanted to get at what it
felt like. He said, "I don't
really think about dying. I
take one day at a time." I
realized then that you go
on living till you're dead.
Life may be compro-
mised, but there's a way
to go on living. You don't
die until you're dead.

– Judy

IF YOU ARE FEELING angry and put-upon, or consumed by thoughts of cancer and treatment, or having difficulty dealing with the demands of the people around you, try to do at least one nice thing for yourself every day. It can be a tiny thing or something loud and noticeable. You are limited only by your imagination. In case your imagination is on the back burner at the moment because of all the rest of the stuff happening in your life right now, here are some suggestions.

- Take a walk each day (it doesn't matter if you can only make it around the house or down the block), or go for a swim if you are well enough. It will do wonders for your morale.

- Enjoy nature.

- If you don't live with children, talk to a small child. Small children can usually remind you of the other world out there, the noncancer one.

- If you do live with children, give yourself a little break. Ask someone to sit with them while you do something for yourself. Or take your children somewhere special.

- Write a letter to your child or children, a letter that can be given to them when they grow up.

- If you feel you need a rest from your emotions for a while, ask your doctor for some medication. Or seek counseling.

- Give yourself a goal for the end of treatment. I got through my course of treatment by planning an exotic holiday. One woman I talked to planned to renovate her kitchen. There are less expensive goals to imagine than these, of course.

- Buy something brightly colored: earrings, a scarf, a flower. Then wear it.

- Rent a humorous video. Laughter is the best stress-reliever.

It may be different for others, but pain is what it took to teach me to pay attention. In times of pain, when the future is too terrifying to contemplate and the past too painful to remember, I have learned to pay attention to right now. The precise moment I was in was always the only safe place for me. Each moment, taken alone, was always bearable. In the exact now, we are all, always, all right. Yesterday the marriage may have ended. Tomorrow the cat may die. The phone call from the lover, for all my waiting, may not ever come, but just at the moment, just now, that's all right. I am breathing in and out. Realizing this, I began to notice that each moment was not without its beauty.

— Julia Cameron,
The Artist's Way

One of the lines I came up with was that in my whirlwind life I didn't take a vacation, so my immune system did. I was doing too many things and needed to devote more time to looking after myself. I decided to set aside one day of the week to do that, and the rest of the time I wouldn't think about cancer. So every Thursday I would go to relaxation group in the morning, have lunch and chitchat with a friend, go to a support group in the afternoon, then to the clinic library where I'd look at videos, audio-tapes, books, everything they had. I did Thursdays like that for about six months, and I usually managed to focus the energies on that day. The rest of the week I just did everything else.

– *Carol*

- Listen to some music you love.

- If chemo has made you bald, paint your head with face paint or makeup.

- Read travel brochures.

- Call a friend you haven't talked to in a while. Or write a letter.

- Rest for an hour on your bed without feeling guilty.

List your own ideas.

Is there something you have always wanted to do, ever since you can remember? Or is there somewhere you want to go for a special vacation? What if this were the last day of your life – how would you most like to spend it? This is not an invitation to be morbid. Just try to imagine what unfinished business you might have to complete. Would you like to tell someone how much you love them? Is there a special place you would like to visit today? Write down your ideas here. You can come back to this page on days when you need to remember that things will get better. Or you can act today on one of the things on your list.

I am taking care of my mind as well as my body. The health of both are important to me.

Record your dreams here.

RELATIONSHIPS

I try to avoid saying to women I'm talking to about it that you'll get back to normal, because you don't get back to being the way you were before. You're physically changed, but you're psychically changed, too, I think.

– Carol

MANY WOMEN FIND their self-image in tatters or at least seriously disarranged after a diagnosis of breast cancer. Self-confidence can desert you; perhaps you discover you are not who or what you believed you were. Your body has betrayed you and you may be afraid that other people will no longer accept you because you have had cancer. If you have had a mastectomy, it may have been difficult for you to come to terms with having only one breast, or no breasts at all if you had a double mastectomy. You may feel or have felt that somehow you are less of a woman because of the surgery. You will almost certainly find that you have to redefine yourself and, sometimes, your relationships with the people around you.

How have you changed? What is different?

FRIENDS MAY NOT KNOW how to talk to you about your diagnosis. While some will be relieved if you make the first move to break the barrier, others won't be able to handle it at all and may stay away from you completely. (As a bonus, you can also use your illness as an excuse not to see people you don't want to see.)

Although you may feel otherwise, it never occurred to me not to talk about my illness to my friends and family. In fact, I was obsessed with it. I tried to be sensitive enough to talk about something else if people didn't want to hear about it. To me, of course, it was the most interesting thing in the world, so I found it difficult to be in social situations while I was going through treatment and for a few months afterward. Everything else seemed artificial, and I found myself incapable of making small talk. Going to support groups gave me the outlet and perspective I needed, and it also helped me to rebuild my self-confidence. However, support groups are not for everyone. Some people fear that other people's painful experiences will overwhelm them, as the following comments of Joan D and Angie demonstrate.

"I didn't want support groups. I wanted something more positive. Right now you have to think, This is my problem, and blank out other people's in order to get well. I used to worry about everybody, but I've learned to keep on an even plane. I can't deal with their problems, and I think a support group would be like that."
   – Joan D

"Going to the support group at the B.C. Cancer Agency made me sadder than I thought. People were supportive, but I found that I took on other people's sorrow, so I would come home not just feeling extremely sad and anxious about my own situation but about theirs, as well. So though it was good to talk to other women, I did wonder sometimes if it wasn't making me more sad than if I hadn't gone. It depended on who was in the group. I found it better to talk to people who had had their diagnosis a year ago or longer, because they had some perspective."
   – Angie

Have you been to a support group? How did you react? Was it helpful?

My view of my body
didn't really change. I
have big boobs, and all it
did was take me down
one cup size. I wish
they'd done the other
side, as well! Because
I've been at home for a
year and a half and I've
been wearing sweatshirts
and so on, I haven't had
to put on real clothes for
so long. I don't feel I've
been part of the real
world, so I'm not exactly
sure what it's going to
feel like when I have to
do that. I think it's going
to make a difference, but
I'm not sure.

– Lynda

Who is particularly important to you right now?

I didn't like being without hair, looking egglike in every way. I was very self-conscious, even more so in England. I remember going into a pub and there were some rowdy people in there. I had a scarf on and someone started taunting me about looking like a gypsy. I got irrationally upset about it. It didn't make any difference in close relationships. That was helpful, and kept my confidence going a bit.

— *Joan A*

I didn't become a different person, but I wasn't the person I had been before, and my partner was comfortable with that person but not comfortable with the person who was going through all this. I needed his support and it wasn't there. He wasn't very willing to talk about it, and certainly not willing to have me joke about it, which was one way I had of coping. He needed to control it, I think, and this was something he couldn't control. It wasn't in his grand plan for himself to be caught up in this kind of stuff. So I just said, "I can't. I haven't got time. I don't know if I'm going to be alive in two days, so get out. Let me concentrate on me."

– *Carol*

Is there anyone you would like to shout or throw rotten eggs at? Write them a letter. Let it all hang out, but don't send it, whatever you do! Write it in this book and leave it here.

My husband didn't usually go with me for treatment, but I have a good friend who used to go with me every time. She was a terrific help. In a way I preferred her going with me rather than him. I didn't want to have to worry about him getting upset or worried, which would be an extra burden for me. After we got the diagnosis, we went out for a walk and he broke down in tears. He felt he couldn't cope or manage the children if I didn't recover. I think he felt very threatened by it, and I found him hard to deal with at times. They really didn't think there was more than a fifty-fifty chance I would recover, and he would start thinking ahead about how he would do things if I were not there. I found that very unhelpful and hurtful. It was a natural reaction on his part – he was terrified. But he was very supportive for the most part.

– Joan A

Did anyone drop out of your life? If so, how do you feel about it?   *Relationships*

161

He's actually been very good. After my surgery, he wanted to check my incision every day to make sure it was okay and not infected. The kids did, too, so it was very much a family thing, not hidden. He looks at it once in a while but never makes negative com- ments, which helps. He's always left the medical aspects of everything to me because I'm a nurse, so this is another thing I'll look after. He'll be there for emotional sup- port, but damned if he's going to read anything about breast cancer.

– Debbie

Do any of your family or friends treat you differently since your diagnosis? How do you feel about that?

I have a pretty supportive group of friends who were willing to talk about it, who didn't feel sorry for me, who were shocked. I immediately saw "I could be next" cross their faces, and a lot of them got mammograms on account of that, women who hadn't thought of it before. Aside from my mother, I didn't experience people not being able to deal with the information. I've heard from other women that they had difficulty with friends who were scared. It is scary for people.

– Carol

My partner has been very supportive. She's not the least bit medically oriented, but she's become very proficient at emptying drains and changing dressings. She was forced to take vacation days after my surgery so as to be at home until the drain came out. It's been very hard for her. One of my brothers was absolutely stupendous. The day I had surgery he took the day off work and came down at 8:00 a.m. and stayed with my partner. He has the weakest stomach going, but when I barfed he was there, emptying basins. Later on he helped me wash my hair and get dressed. He took me out for lunch. Anything I wanted, he did. He's been absolutely wonderful and good support for my partner. He said they had lots of nice

talks and he took her out for lunch and insisted on paying. My mother collapsed at the diagnosis, which came six weeks after her husband's death. She couldn't face that. She did bring meals down, though she wouldn't stay.
– *Elaine*

IF YOU ARE A WOMAN who doesn't have a partner, you may have decided that a romantic relationship is the last thing you want when you are dealing with cancer, and you may have put that side of your social life on hold in order to concentrate on getting well. Meanwhile, all around you, people are meeting, falling in love, falling out of love. Even if you cannot imagine it now, you will eventually be brave enough to take part again in what the rest of the world has been doing while you have been away. Perhaps your self-confidence has taken a nosedive and the new you isn't sure how to go out and meet the world again. If you have had a mastectomy, you may be unsure about how to relate to the world as a one-breasted woman. Or you may just decide that you have had it with romance and want to live your life differently.

At the risk of sounding like a broken record, I will repeat that support groups can help you to find your footing again. Or you could see a counselor. There are several helpful books, too: by far the best I found is *Spinning Straw into Gold: Your Emotional Recovery from Breast Cancer* by Ronnie Kaye. She has been there, and she knows what it is like.

IT IS NOT JUST the patient who experiences breast cancer; the family is deeply involved, as well. In fact, it may be even more difficult for families to live with the diagnosis than it is for the patient. While some families are accustomed to sharing concerns and fears and are open to listening to one another, others don't communicate quite so extensively or easily. Then there are families who don't believe that talking about such things is helpful at all.

Where does your family fit in? Have you found it easy or difficult to talk about your concerns?

My daughter, who was 11, knew there was a chance I might not recover. She was going through a terrible stage herself, just getting epilepsy, and had been given the wrong medication. She was throwing temper tantrums and was too busy with herself to take much notice of it and a bit jealous that I was getting more attention than she was. Ben [five] was my lifeline really. He was such a merry little boy, and I felt I really wanted to see him grow up. When he first saw me without the wig and without the scarf, he said, "Oh, you've got nice ears." I thought, Wow! That's really nice. He wasn't frightened at all. I thought he might be, but I don't think he understood the implications.

– Joan A

My first reaction when I got the news was that I wouldn't be able to tell my mother. I was right. She was extremely upset and unable to talk about it at all. It was hard for her. Cancer for that generation is a death sentence. She didn't know how to talk about it, and I didn't know how to help her. Maybe I was angry myself, and trying to cope with my partner and my mother at the same time was too much.

– Carol

PARENTS TEND TO give preschoolers simple explanations about illness, believing that they are too young to understand it fully. Young school-aged children may feel scared and lonely, and may even believe that mom is sick because of something they did. Older children who are still at school can be preoccupied with their own lives and resent the disruption cancer brings to the household. Adolescent daughters can have a particularly difficult time; they are expected to help more around the house and are sometimes aware that they might be at risk themselves. Some daughters start doing regular breast self-examinations; others aren't interested. Some women take their children along once or twice when they are going to be examined by the surgeon or oncologist, or when they are going to have chemo or radiation treatments. If a child can actually be there with you, she or he is less likely to imagine the worst when you go off on your own for appointments.

Has your partner (if you have one) been able to communicate his or her fears to you? If you have children, or if there are children close to you, how have they reacted?

To be sick or disfigured is one thing, but to have teenagers at the same time is another. They are self-centered and they love you incredibly, but you are also their support system in every way. My daughter is a very intense kid. She worries about a lot of things and takes on a lot of things. . . . My husband kept a journal as a way of dealing with it. I don't think men articulate these things very well, and he was the receptacle for me unloading tons of fear and emotion for months on end. Men are brought up to believe that they should look after their wives physically and emotionally, and if they love them as well, they want to take care of them. It's terrible to sit by and watch somebody you love go through something like that. He developed support at

work, but you're not
going to sit down as a
grown man in your office
and cry on somebody's
shoulder. Not usually. I
don't think it's healthy
for men [not to be able to
show their feelings].
— *Angie*

*I am taking care of myself first and
foremost. I am coping with my family
and friends the best way I can.*

Record your dreams here.

BODY IMAGE AND SEXUALITY

Body image and sexuality are issues of concern for everybody. People don't always talk about these topics, because often there are other things they are more concerned about, such as: "Is this treatment going to work? Am I going to survive? Am I going to have support around me?" Yet the themes of body image and sexuality are important, and they relate to the question: "Am I still going to be lovable?" It's important to talk about it. A support group can be particularly helpful for dealing with body image and sexuality, in revealing that other people are often facing similar thoughts, and in providing creative responses and solutions from other members. Group discussions can come alive with humor, which breaks the tension and can be a wonderful coping device. . . . Acknowledging the problems is an important step in coping with them.

– Dr. Elaine Drysdale

WHILE MANY WOMEN are afraid that their altered appearance will make them unattractive to their partners, or that their partners will leave them because they have cancer, single women often fear that they will never be able to attract anyone again.

How do you feel about your body now? Have your feelings changed? If you have a partner, have you been able to talk with him or her about it? If you don't have a partner, have you been able or wanted to talk with anyone about it?

As Ronnie Kaye says in her marvelous book *Spinning Straw into Gold*: "In general, I find that men come through beautifully, if we let them. Unfortunately, when women send out signals about how terrible they feel, and how they don't want to be seen, much less touched, men may back off for fear of hurting or embarrassing their partners. Women can misinterpret that as a message about how unacceptable they are. . . . It is unrealistic to expect a man to have no reaction whatsoever to the fact that his wife or lover has lost a breast. Breasts are a lovely part of an intimate relationship, bringing pleasure to both partners. It is quite appropriate for a man to feel a real sense of loss should his partner lose one or both of her breasts. However, a truly intimate relationship hinges on far more than a woman's breasts. Most of the men I have spoken to tell me that any loss they may feel is temporary, and they are much more concerned with their partner's life than with her breast(s). If it is hard for a woman to confront her altered appearance for the first time, her partner deserves some latitude as well. It's not fair to expect a man to adjust to a significant change in his partner's body and feel sexual all at the same time. When a woman is having difficulty showing her partner her surgery, I will recommend that they find a place away from the bedroom where they can help each other discuss, look, and touch in a completely nonsexual way. That way, they can become reacquainted as they both adapt to the changes in her body."

Perhaps you can identify with some of the following comments:

"I'm not embarrassed about my body image. I still feel like the same person. Being alive and able to get back doing things outweighed the importance of having body parts missing."
– Brenda

"After the mastectomy, it took me a long time to get casual about it, and in mixed settings I still feel shy."
– Jo

"The whole experience has a great impact on confidence. Your body is out of control. Some women like how they look with reconstruc-

tion and some women have a decreased interest in sex. It can have an impact with a regular partner. Women don't feel like being the nurturing one. They may want to be nurtured themselves. They can be physically intimate but not wear themselves out. For single women the problem can be how to introduce the subject."

— Elizabeth Dohan

"I talked with my friends, and we joked about it. My sister-in-law wrote to me about a friend of hers who had a false boob that you blew up like a balloon. It escaped and flew up to the ceiling. We laughed and laughed."

— Adine

"I've never had a concept of myself as someone with a body beautiful, a ravishing individual. I've always defined myself more by what I'm able to do. Contrary to popular belief, my sexuality is not attached to the outside of my chest wall. . . . My one concern about whether I wanted to have the second mastectomy was that one of the things my partner says attracted her to me was my large-bustedness. When I asked her about the second surgery, she said, 'It's your decision.' And when I finally announced that I was going ahead with it, she just sat there and said, 'Thank God. That's what I wanted you to do all along.' We're just going to find all these ways of deriving pleasure, like going on a second honeymoon. It's exciting."

— Elaine

"I wanted to have sex when I was in the 'abyss.' I wanted to feel close and connected to my partner, and alive. There was no enjoyment about it, just to be as close as possible, connecting with his soul. Being held and touched was more important in the beginning — it had to do with not dying."

— Judy

"It's hard to feel sexy when you are throwing up and bald."
— *Dr. Susan Love's Breast Book*

CHEMOTHERAPY CAN AFFECT how a woman feels about her body and her sexuality, and many women find themselves unsure whether what they are feeling is caused by chemo or chemo-induced menopause. Radiation can cause fatigue, and depression can affect a woman's sex drive. The experts say these feelings are usually temporary and that things gradually return to normal. The best thing to do is to communicate your needs to your partner: if all you want is to be hugged from time to time, your partner will probably be glad to know that and will be able to feel helpful.

Sometimes a relationship or marriage that might be heading for the rocks founders when the stress of a cancer diagnosis and treatment is added to it. Women often decide to leave an unhealthy relationship that may have been causing them stress for a long time. Or they may find an opportunity to reexamine the relationship. It isn't always easy to communicate feelings at the best of times, but it is especially important when it *isn't* the best of times.

It wasn't until I took off my wig for the last time that I felt I was really me again. While I was still wearing it, I remember standing in a supermarket lineup and being aware that a man standing in another lineup was looking at me admiringly. As I wrote in my diary at the time, I was outraged: "There's no point in my even looking back at him, is there? What am I going to say: 'Hi, my name's Jennifer and I'm having chemotherapy for cancer right now'? Can't think what he could have been doing looking at me, anyway, not the way I look. He must have been desperate." When I did finally decide to stop wearing even scarves or a hat, let alone the wig, it was a huge relief. My hair was less than an inch long, and I looked as if I was making a fashion statement, although I was a bit old to be trying to cultivate the punk look. But I didn't care. I finally felt I could face the world as myself for the first time in months.

Write down your own concerns and experiences concerning body image and sexuality. Everyone reacts in a different way. Whatever your feelings are, they are yours to be honored and acknowledged.

I honor my body as much as my soul.
They both deserve love and attention.

Record your dreams here.

WHERE DO I GO FROM HERE?

It felt as if I had completed an obstacle course, or run a race. Now the finish line had been reached and I wondered what direction I should take from here to live the long, healthy, and active life I wanted.

– Judy

TREATMENT IS OVER. You are probably having regular checkups, but essentially you are now on your own. Perhaps you are taking tamoxifen for the next few years. Whatever the case, you are out of the acute stage.

If this is the end of treatment for you, the first thing to do is congratulate yourself for having come through it. You did it! You may not have thought you could, but you did. And believe it or not, there will come a time when cancer is no longer the first thing you think of when you wake up in the morning.

Here is how I felt:

"Last radiation treatment today! It was done by two technologists I hadn't seen before, but they seemed pleasant enough. It would have been nice if someone had been there to help mark the end of treatment: someone to shake my hand at the very least and say, 'Well done. You came through it.' It seemed very hollow to walk out of the building by myself, without anything to mark the occasion. I'm too tired even to cry, so I went to the beach, walked a little, and sat on a log till I felt calmer. A beautiful bunch of flowers arrived from Julie as congratulations for finishing treatment. They're absolutely lovely: bright red, yellow, and blue. Cheered me up no end."
  – from my own diary, September 1993

HERE IS WHAT others have to say about the completion of treatment:

"I think what happens is that for the first few months people are very solicitous. Your friends are all around you, the medical community is there, you are actually in treatment. Then it finishes, and people go on asking you for a while how you're feeling. Then you start to pick up and people stop talking about it – they think you're going to be okay. I found that for about three months I was angry a lot of the time, and I was depressed and not picking up."
  – Angie

"You just have to look ahead and not get too anxious. A lot of recovery is positive thinking, or looking ahead and not dwelling on the

cancer. You have to be sensible about it. After all, I could have been run over by a truck all these years [since she was diagnosed in 1971]."

— Adine

"Initially there can be a whirlwind of activity related to treatment. In addition to numerous medical appointments and procedures, people often go to naturopaths, wellness groups, relaxation sessions, et cetera. When the appointments taper down and a woman's energy is no longer so directed toward external events, there can be a sense of shock or even abandonment. Then the impact of cancer can hit. It is important to talk about feelings, to look at getting on with life, and to look at whatever issue is germane for that person. Often people have been so busy through treatment that they have put an issue on hold, such as a dysfunctional marital relationship, only to have to face it later. After the active treatment has ended, people often ask such questions as: 'Should I end this relationship now or not? What should I do with my life? Should I go back to that job that I never liked, anyway? Are my values and priorities different now?'. . . I think that having cancer can be a real wake-up call for some people."

— Dr. Elaine Drysdale

"Women can fall into low-level depression after treatment, waiting for it [cancer] to come back. I tell them they're not alone in that. It's perfectly natural."
— *Dr. A. W. Tolcher.*

YOU MAY CHOOSE to get counseling. Continuing to use relaxation, meditation, and visualizations can help. Some women also use the Internet as a way to keep in touch with other women with breast cancer and to discuss their concerns and fears with them. The Internet also provides another way to keep up with the latest breast cancer research from around the world.

I recently took a course in Chi gong, an ancient Oriental healing art combining mental concentration and breathing exercises, which has helped me to keep focused on what I need to do. I also attend, although not regularly, a support group that usually invites a speaker for part of the evening. One month the speaker was a breast cancer surgeon who explained all kinds of helpful stuff about axillary dissection (taking lymph nodes out of the armpit).

I started going to the group a year after I'd finished all the treatment. It was at that point I felt I needed to look back and reflect on it. Up till then I had enough support around me that I didn't need outside support.

– Lynda

Some women say that having cancer is the best thing that ever happened to them. They say it kick-started them out of the rut in which they had been stuck. Because they don't know how much time they may have left, they want to make the most of whatever time they do have. Others say it is the worst thing that ever happened to them. It is probably a bit of both. Enjoying your life is important, but it is also important not to feel guilty if you don't want to make huge changes to your life just yet, if ever. It is impossible for most of us to live every second of every day as if it were our last; the occasional pause to admire a sunset or a flower can be enough to keep us going.

Were you stuck in some area of your life before the cancer diagnosis? If so, has that changed? Do you want it to change?

Did you make any promises to yourself while you were going through treatment? Did you make resolutions or set goals for yourself? If you did, what were they? Is it realistic for you to expect to achieve all of them? Which ones can you achieve?

It gets to be a part of you, whatever you had done, I think. Think of the people walking around with only one leg, or no eyes. I think you have to get away from the constant awareness. They wanted me to go to a group, but I didn't think I could cope with other people so I said no. I hardly thought about it after three or four years, though it's still irritating when I try to get a decent bathing suit.

– Adine

MOST OF THE WOMEN I interviewed haven't made any enormous changes in their lives:

> *"It's all moments, isn't it? You have acute peaks – you're on that edge, with a heightened awareness of your surroundings. When you're back in the groove, the old baggage is picked up. At the job I used to be very critical of myself. Now I just try to reframe it and throw it back out into the universe."*
>
> – Judy

> *"When I finished radiation, I had three goals. I wanted to try to get fit again. I wanted to lose 10 pounds – everything I read talked about a high-fat diet and I began to wonder if cancer wasn't associated with weight somehow. I wanted to feel safer. And I wanted to get back to work because I'd been at home for about six months and thought it would be better to have a focus outside of my family. So now I'm back in a very busy state again, and although we talked a lot about stopping to smell the roses, I think I'm busier now than I ever was. It scares me sometimes."*
>
> – Angie

> *"I like my life. I see what they mean about life never being the same afterward, but I wish I didn't have to go through this kind of torment. An innocent person shouldn't have to go through this, taking it like punishment. It's like you're testing yourself: 'I'll be really, really good and it won't come back, and Teacher won't spank me.' Just like a little girl."*
>
> – Joan D

> *"I figure the main lesson I've learned is to be more moderate. My rehab counselor is watching that. Am I going to moderate my life-style and work habits, or am I going to jump back into the old ways? When you've had to take a year and a half out of your life, it's a fairly significant thing to remember. And I do think I'll be a lot better on the whole. . . . I painted at school and am quite creative. I like doing that kind of stuff, and I have a painting collage in*

my mind. *I'm not good at it, but I do it. I did two paintings between mammogram and biopsy and biopsy and surgery, and it's interesting because the one before the biopsy is all soft waves and pastel colors. And then afterward there was all this brightly charged electric stuff that's red and orange and gold."*

– Lynda

"I'm still not doing what I want to do when I grow up. I went and got my oil paints out again and am starting to learn how to relax by painting. I'm putting my energies into something pleasurable. Before anything happens again I want to learn about myself. I'm living on the edge of never knowing. There's a lot of guessing going on in the science of dealing with cancer. You'd think there would be more people with answers."

– Val

"The longer it is after surgery, the easier it is to slip back into the old ways, and it grieves me when I do that. I promised I'd take the time to relax and enjoy the world, but the world catches up with you and you slip back into it. You start losing the hard-won realizations you had about yourself."

– Jo

"Find some particular thing your soul craves for nourishment and do it."
– Audre Lorde, A Burst of Light

AS DR. ELAINE DRYSDALE SAYS: "For some people, recovery after cancer can bring a dramatic change in perspective, somewhat like a religious conversion. They may experience a sudden shift in values and the thrill of appreciating life anew. This can settle into a quieter, less obvious kind of outlook in which the changes become incorporated into the person's approach to life generally. People who were initially ecstatic, saying, 'Look at the trees, look at the flowers,' may be slightly less vocal about their appreciation a few years later, but they probably have a much deeper respect for the beauty of life than they had prior to the cancer. With time the appreciation becomes more integrated, more subtle."

How do you feel about your life and about the life around you now?

I WILL ALWAYS REMEMBER a visit shortly after my surgery from a man I know from my business life who had had colon cancer about a year before. He asked how I was really feeling (only someone who has had cancer knows how to ask that question), then talked about his own experience. He told me that you have to view each day as a gift and live accordingly. What impressed me most was that he said he had looked at his life to see if there was anything he wanted to change and had decided there wasn't. How wonderful to be able to say that about your own life; I certainly couldn't have said it about mine. What do you know now that you wish you had known when you were first diagnosed?

Imagine that this is the first day of the rest of your life. (It is, if you look at it literally.) How would you like to spend the rest of your life? Be both humorous and serious. List your dreams and fantasies, then set some realistic goals – for six months ahead, for one year, and then for three years from now. (There is a special page for your goals or plans following the blank pages.)

For the next six months:

1.

2.

3.

For one year from now:

1.

2.

3.

For three years from now:

1.

2.

3.

List any additional goals and how you can achieve them.

Record your dreams here.

LIVING WITH CANCER

And did you get what
you wanted from this life, even so?
I did.
And what did you want?
To call myself beloved, to feel myself
beloved on the earth.

– Raymond Carver, "Late Fragment," from
A New Path to the Waterfall

I went to the oncologist and said, "Tell me what to do and I'll do it so cancer won't come back. I don't know what to do. Should I be feeling guilty for eating this or this?" The oncologist said, "Joan, go live. We can't tell you what will bring it back and what won't." So that's what I'm doing.

— *Joan D*

The likelihood of recurrence is greatest within five years. Between five to eight years we approach with optimism. After 10 years recurrence gets increasingly rare. We can't say with certainty that it won't come back. It shakes people to the core.

— *Dr. A. W. Tolcher*

MOST OF US do what we can to keep well: maintain a healthier diet, drink less alcohol, do more exercise, make time to relax and sleep, try to avoid too much stress, and engage in more of the things that we enjoy. But the unpalatable truth we all have to face is that for now breast cancer is not a 100 percent curable disease. About 5,400 women died from breast cancer in Canada in 1995.

Recurrence. There isn't one of us who doesn't think about it, or a new primary cancer developing. For months after my treatment ended I would wake in the middle of the night overcome with terror, convinced that the cells in my body had gone crazy. Almost the only time I feel that way now is the night before I have to go to the clinic for checkups. I have always had trouble pronouncing the word *metastasis*. The trouble is that I don't want to pronounce it at all, as if saying it correctly will cause the cancer to come back, or to spread, which is what the word means. I trust and believe that the anxiety will lessen over time.

Those women who do have recurrences, or cancer developing in the other breast, have a special set of circumstances to face. Dr. Elaine Drysdale says that "Most women react to news of the initial diagnosis of cancer with a sense of shock, but also with a sense of optimism that makes them feel as though they will beat it. A number of women have told me that news of a recurrence was also a shock, but that it was much more difficult this time to generate optimism and faith in their strategies. So with news of a recurrence, there may be slightly less shock but even more anguish."

Many of us become much more aware of our bodies after a diagnosis of cancer, and can be easily panicked when various aches and pains occur. Most pains that come and go quickly are not likely to be cancer, but if you have any persistent symptoms that worry you, you should see your doctor and have them investigated. You are going for regular checkups, as well, so you have your bases covered.

Many recurrences are found by women doing breast self-examination (as are many first tumors). The earlier the tumor is found, the better your chances of survival if it is a local recurrence or a tumor in the opposite breast. If you don't know how to do BSE, there are books that can help. Or you can ask your doctor, or a nurse, or find a teaching clinic. If you do find any worrisome changes, tell your doctor and have them investigated. It is also important not to feel that you have failed somehow if the cancer does come back. You are not to blame; cancer follows no rules that we know about. You have done what you could.

Many of us celebrate anniversaries of the date on which we were diagnosed. My friend Carol is just coming up to the sixth anniversary of her surgery; I have just had my fourth. My friend Jo has been cancer-free for 16 years now, and Adine for 26. Somehow it seems more joyous to celebrate each year of life since illness than to celebrate a birthday. We are all members of what Arthur Frank, author of *The Wounded Storyteller*, calls "the remission society" – people who are, in fact, well but can never be considered to be cured (something like a secret society among people who are healthy). Some of us celebrate our anniversary on the date of surgery, others on the date of diagnosis, and still others on the date when treatment finished. It is up to you! It is your anniversary.

Some of us use the experience of having cancer to turn our energy or leftover anger or outrage to doing volunteer work. We write, counsel others, donate money for research, fund-raise, organize events, lobby politicians for more research money, make ourselves heard. Things have been improving on the breast cancer research front, but much more money is needed. If we are to be heard, we must speak up. We need to make it better for the women who will be diagnosed in the future, and to prod researchers into discovering the cause or causes of the disease so that it can be prevented. Early detection saves lives, no doubt of that, but wouldn't it be better if breast cancer didn't happen in the first place?

Other people want to forget all about the disease and go back to a normal life as soon as they can. Fine, go to it!

There are many ways we refer to ourselves: as cancer survivors, or women who have been treated for cancer, or cancer veterans, or women living with breast cancer. One woman who knew she was unlikely to survive the disease said, "I'm a cancer fighter, not a survivor. I want people to know that." Or we may not want to refer to it at all, which is our perfect right.

Life is now, this minute. What am I waiting for?

It's a shadow over us, for sure, but the upside is that it has made us more grateful for what we have. It sounds like a cliché, but it's absolutely true. It takes a threat to make you appreciate what you've got.

– Angie

I got chest pains after carrying something heavy recently, so I went to the clinic because I was convinced I had cancer growing in my ribs. My GP thought I had pulled ligaments in my chest. I had to wait three weeks for the bone scan. I fretted about it so much that I got a bald patch on my head. It turned out to be okay, though.

– Brenda

Record your dreams and any thoughts you have here.

It came to me that the choice of when I die is not likely to be mine. *Grace and Grit* [by Ken Wilber and Treya Killam Wilber] says that your mental attitude can affect disease, but probably not much more than 20 percent, and what I want to know is if Treya Wilber was such an evolved and compassionate human being who learned to accept what was happening to her, why did the disease take over so completely and give her such a horrible time? Is it true that the more evolved you become, the more you are tested?
— *from my own diary,*
May 1993

For a while I considered some radical diets, whether to plant my entire garden with kale and graze all day. But when you're working, feeding a family, and running a big house, you revert to your old habits. I now eat a really low-fat diet, though.

– Angie

People still don't know that there are many people who are fine after diagnosis and treatment and go on living for a very long time, though they have to be checked up every year. You don't hear the happy stories or the successes. You always hear of the women who died.

– Silvia Wilson

Hope, faith, love, and a
strong will to live offer no
promise of immortality,
only proof of our unique-
ness as human beings
and the opportunity to
experience full growth
even under the grimmest
circumstances. The clock
provides only a technical
measurement of how
long we live. Far more
real than the ticking of
time is the way we open
up the minutes and
invest them with mean-
ing. Death is not the ultimate tragedy in life. The
ultimate tragedy is to die
without discovering the
possibilities of full
growth. The approach of
death need not be denial
of that growth.

— *Norman Cousins,*
Head First

I've never been more optimistic about cancer treatment than I am now. We have to find out what changes inside a cell. It's an exciting time. With the harder cancers we are only getting to the point of understanding the disease in order to change it. The next step is to turn off the faulty gene. With a family history of breast cancer we can identify the genes to be changed. We are reversing genes in animal studies, and we may add medicines to turn down genes. It would be nice to be able to think of cancer in the way we think of TB now.

— *Dr. A. W. Tolcher.*

Whether we come to
realize our illnesses are
accidents of birth, the
result of radiation expo-
sure, God's punishment,
or God's grace, there is
always a teaching to be
found. That does not
necessarily mean that
teaching is the purpose
of illness, or that sick
people are more in need
of that advice, it is just
an inevitable outcome of
the profound transfor-
mations that come with
the territory. . . . Our lives
condense, collapse, and
recoalesce, requiring
changes, and we are
responsible to those
changes. We are not
responsible *for* our illnesses, we are respon-
sible *to* them, to what
they offer and require of
all of us, sick and
well alike.

– Kat Duff,
The Alchemy of Illness

SUGGESTED READING

THE FOLLOWING IS only a partial list of the publications available to women with breast cancer. You will find more at the library, or your local bookstore, and the Cancer Information Service (1-888-939-3333) can tell you about others. I found the works marked with an asterisk particularly useful.

ABOUT CANCER AND BREAST CANCER

Anderson, Greg. *50 Essential Things to Do When the Doctor Says It's Cancer*. New York: Plume, 1993.

Atlantic Breast Cancer Information Project. *Breast Cancer: Questions You Might Want to Ask*. Charlottetown, PEI, 1995. Available from Breast Cancer Information Exchange Projects (see Breast Cancer Information Projects in "Other Resources" for contact information).

* Austin, Steve, and Cathy Hitchcock. *Breast Cancer: What You Should Know (but May Not Be Told) About Prevention, Diagnosis and Treatment*. Rocklin, CA: Prima Publishing, 1994.

* Batt, Sharon. *Patient No More: The Politics of Breast Cancer*. Charlottetown, PEI: Gynergy Books, 1994.

Braddock, Suzanne, et al. *Straight Talk About Breast Cancer*. Omaha: Addicus Books, 1994.

Breast Cancer Action. *Lymphedema: A Breast Cancer Legacy*. Ottawa, 1996. Available for $2 from Breast Cancer Action Ottawa, Billings Bridge Plaza, P.O. Box 39041, Ottawa, Ontario KIA IAI. Phone: (613) 736-5921.

* Bruning, Nancy. *Coping with Chemotherapy*. 1985. New York: Ballantine, 1993.

* Buckman, Robert. *What You Really Need to Know About Cancer: A Comprehensive Guide for Patients and Their Families*. Toronto: Key Porter and the Canadian Cancer Society, 1995.

* Burlington Breast Cancer Support Services. *What You Need to Know About Breast Cancer: A Booklet for Women with Breast Cancer and Those Who Care About Them*. Burlington, ON, 1996. Available from Breast Cancer Information Exchange Projects (see Breast Cancer Information Projects in "Other Resources" for contact information). This publication also contains an excellent list of national and international sources of information, support, and advocacy.

Dollinger, Malin, Ernest H. Rosenbaum, and Greg Cable. *Everyone's Guide to Cancer Therapy: How Cancer Is Diagnosed, Treated, and Managed Day to Day*. Toronto: Somerville House, 1992.

Engel, June. *The Complete Breast Book*. Toronto: Key Porter, 1996.

Johnson, Judi, and Linda Klein. *I Can Cope: Staying Healthy with Cancer*. Minneapolis: Chronimed Publishing, 1994.

* Komarnicky, Lydia, Anne Rosenberg, and Marian Betancourt. *What to Do If You Get Breast Cancer*. Boston: Little, Brown, 1995.

LaTour, Kathy. *The Breast Cancer Companion: From Diagnosis Through Treatment to Recovery, Everything You Need to Know for Every Step Along the Way*. New York: William Morrow, 1994.

* Love, Susan M., and Karen Lindsey. *Dr. Susan Love's Breast Book*. 2nd ed. Menlo Park, CA: Addison-Wesley, 1995.

McKay, Judith, and Nancee Hirano. *The Chemotherapy Survival Guide: Information, Suggestions and Support to Help You Get Through Chemotherapy*. Oakland, CA: New Harbinger, 1993.

* Olivotto, Ivo, Karen Gelmon, and Urve Kuusk. *Breast Cancer: All You Need to Know to Take an Active Part in Your Treatment*. Vancouver: Intelligent Patient Guides, 1995.

Stumm, Diana. *Recovering from Breast Surgery: Exercises to Strengthen Your Body and Relieve Pain*. Alameda, CA: Hunter House, 1995.

COMPLEMENTARY OR ALTERNATIVE THERAPIES

Benjamin, Harold. *The Wellness Community Guide to Fighting for Recovery from Cancer*. New York: Putnam, 1995. (Revised and expanded edition of *From Victim to Victor*.)

Benson, Herbert. *The Relaxation Response*. New York: William Morrow, 1975.

Burton Goldberg Group. *Alternative Medicine: The Definitive Guide*. Puyallup, WA: Future Medicine Publishing, 1994.

Cousins, Norman. *Head First: The Biology of Hope and the Healing Power of the Human Spirit*. New York: Dutton/Signet-Penguin, 1990.

Dong, Paul, and Aristide H. Esser. *Chi Gong: The Ancient Chinese Way to Health*. New York: Marlowe, 1990.

Fontana, David. *The Meditator's Handbook: A Comprehensive Guide to Eastern and Western Meditation Techniques*. Rockport, MA: Element, 1992.

Fugh-Berman, Adriane. *Alternative Medicine: What Works*. Tucson: Odonian Press, 1996.

Garfield, Patricia. *Creative Dreaming*. New York: Ballantine, 1985.

———. *The Healing Power of Dreams*. New York: Simon and Schuster, 1991.

Gawain, Shakti. *Creative Visualization: Use the Power of Your Imagination to Create What You Want in Your Life*. San Rafael, CA: New World Library, 1995.

———. *Meditations: Creative Visualizations and Meditation Exercises to Enrich Your Life*. San Rafael, CA: New World Library, 1991.

Kabat-Zinn, Jon. *Full Catastrophe Living: Using the Wisdom of Your Body and Mind to Face Stress, Pain and Illness.* New York: Delta Books, 1990.

Kushi, Michio, and Alex Jack. *The Cancer Prevention Diet.* Rev. ed. New York: St. Martin's Press, 1993.

Lasater, Judith. *Relax and Renew: Restful Yoga for Stressful Times.* Berkeley: Rodmell Press, 1995.

* Lerner, Michael. *Choices in Healing: Integrating the Best of Conventional and Complementary Approaches to Cancer.* Cambridge, MA: MIT Press, 1994.

Masters, Robert, and Jean Houston. *Mind Games.* New York: Dorset Press, 1990.

Ontario Breast Cancer Information Exchange Project. *A Guide to Unconventional Cancer Therapies.* Toronto, 1994. To order: Write, call, or fax R & R Bookbar, 14800 Yonge Street, Unit 106, Aurora, Ontario L4G 1N3. Phone: (905) 727-3300. Fax: (905) 727-2620.

Pelton, Ross, and Lee Overholser. *Alternatives in Cancer Therapy: The Complete Guide to Non-Traditional Treatments.* New York: Simon and Schuster, 1994.

* Siegel, Bernie S. *Love, Medicine and Miracles: Lessons Learned About Self-Healing from a Surgeon's Experience with Exceptional Patients.* New York: HarperCollins, 1986. (Also available on CD-ROM.)

————. *Peace, Love and Healing.* New York: HarperCollins, 1986.

Simonton, O. Carl, Stephanie Matthews-Simonton, and James Creighton. *Getting Well Again.* New York: Bantam, 1978.

Weller, Stella. *Yoga Therapy: Safe, Natural Methods to Promote Healing and Restore Health and Well-Being.* London: Thorsons, 1995.

Information packages on various complementary therapies are also available through the Cancer Information Service (1-888-939-3333). They are compiled by the Canadian Breast Cancer Research Initiative.

Butler, Sandra, and Barbara Rosenblum. *Cancer in Two Voices.* San Francisco: Spinsters Book Company, 1991.

Cousins, Norman. *Anatomy of an Illness as Perceived by the Patient: Reflections on Healing and Regeneration.* New York: Norton, 1979.

* Dackman, Linda. *Up Front: Sex and the Post-Mastectomy Woman.* New York: Viking, 1990.

Frank, Arthur W. *The Wounded Storyteller: Body, Illness, and Ethics.* Chicago: University of Chicago Press, 1995.

Hart, Judy. *Love, Judy: Letters of Hope and Healing for Women with Breast Cancer.* Berkeley: Conari Press, 1993.

Lorde, Audre. *Cancer Journals.* San Francisco: Aunt Lute Books, 1980.

MacPhee, Rosalind. *Picasso's Woman.* Vancouver: Douglas and McIntyre, 1994.

Moch, Susan Diemert. *Breast Cancer: Twenty Women's Stories.* New York: National League for Nursing, 1995.

Wadler, Joyce. *My Breast: One Woman's Cancer Story.* Reading, MA: Addison-Wesley, 1992.

* Wilber, Ken. *Grace and Grit: Spirituality and Healing in the Life and Death of Treya Killam Wilber.* Boston: Shambhala Publications, 1991.

Williams, Penelope. *That Other Place: A Personal Account of Breast Cancer.* Toronto: Dundurn Press, 1993.

Wittman, Juliet. *Breast Cancer Journal: A Century of Petals.* Golden, CO: Fulcrum, 1993.

Anderson, Greg. *The 22 (Non-Negotiable) Laws of Wellness*. San Francisco: Harper San Francisco, 1995.

Buckman, Robert. *I Don't Know What to Say: How to Help and Support Someone Who Is Dying*. Toronto: Key Porter, 1988.

Dackman, Linda. *Affirmations, Meditations, and Encouragements for Women Living with Breast Cancer*. Los Angeles: Lowell House, 1991; San Francisco: Harper San Francisco, 1992.

Duff, Kat. *The Alchemy of Illness*. New York: Pantheon, 1993.

Fiore, Neil A. *The Road Back to Health: Coping with the Emotional Side of Cancer*. New York: Bantam, 1984.

* Kaye, Ronnie. *Spinning Straw into Gold: Your Emotional Recovery from Breast Cancer*. New York: Simon and Schuster, 1991.

Kübler-Ross, Elisabeth. *On Death and Dying*. New York: Macmillan, 1969.

Moore, Thomas. *Care of the Soul: A Guide for Cultivating Depth and Sacredness in Everyday Life*. New York: HarperCollins, 1992.

Moyers, Bill. *Healing and the Mind*. New York: Doubleday, 1993.

Murcia, Andy. *Man to Man: When the Woman You Love Has Breast Cancer*. New York: St. Martin's Press, 1990.

Schlessel Harpham, Wendy. *After Cancer: A Guide to Your New Life*. 1994. New York: Harper Perennial, 1995.

Siegel, Bernie S. *How to Live Between Office Visits*. New York: HarperCollins, 1993.

Sontag, Susan. *Illness as Metaphor*. 1978. New York: Farrar, Straus and Giroux, 1988.

* Spiegel, David. *Living Beyond Limits: New Hope and Help for Facing Life-Threatening Illness*. New York: Random House, 1993.

Goodman, Michelle. *Vanishing Cookies: Doing OK When a Parent Has Cancer.* Downsview, ON: Benjamin Institute for Community Education and Referral, 1990.

Schaefer, Dan, and Christine Lyons. *How Do We Tell the Children?* New York: Newmarket Press, 1993.

ABOUT WRITING AND JOURNAL WRITING

Baldwin, Christina. *Life's Companion: Journal Writing as a Spiritual Quest.* New York: Bantam, 1991.

* Cameron, Julia. *The Artist's Way: A Spiritual Path to Higher Creativity.* New York: Tarcher-Putnam, 1992.

Lamott, Anne. *Bird by Bird: Some Instructions on Writing and Life.* New York: Pantheon Books, 1994.

Progoff, Ira. *At a Journal Workshop.* New York: Dialogue House Library, 1975.

* Rainer, Tristine. *The New Diary.* Los Angeles: Jeremy P. Tarcher, 1978.

Schiwy, Marlene. *A Voice of Her Own: Women and the Journal-Writing Journey.* New York: Simon and Schuster, 1996.

OTHER RESOURCES

Booklets are available from your nearest Canadian Cancer Society office, or the Breast Cancer Information Projects listed below. Local support groups, cancer hospitals, and treatment centers usually have helpful videos, pamphlets, or booklets, as do some surgeons' and physicians' offices. Some material is also available in other languages.

Across Canada contact: Cancer Information Service and Breast Cancer Information Project at 1-888-939-3333. This service is given under the auspices of the Canadian Cancer Society, with information from the B.C. Cancer Agency's breast cancer specialists.

The Canadian Cancer Society runs a volunteer visitor program. You will be able to ask questions of and discuss your experiences with a woman who has had breast cancer. Call the society office nearest to you.

The Canadian Breast Cancer Foundation's *Breast Cancer Resource Handbook* lists agencies and organizations that provide emotional and psychological support. Call your local office of the foundation for a copy.

The First Nations Breast Cancer Society can be contacted at: Box 14, 415 West Esplanade, North Vancouver, British Columbia. v7m 1a6. Phone: (604) 876-0675. Website: *www.uniserve.com/lifeenergy/breastcancer/breast.html*

BREAST CANCER INFORMATION PROJECTS

Atlantic Breast Cancer Information Project
c/o Canadian Cancer Society, P.E.I. Division
P.O. Box 115
Charlottetown, Prince Edward Island C1A 7K2
Phone: (902) 892-9531 or (902) 566-4007. Fax: (902) 628-8281

B.C. and Yukon Breast Cancer Information Project
c/o Canadian Cancer Society, B.C. and Yukon Division
565 West 10th Avenue
Vancouver, British Columbia V5Z 4J4
Phone: (604) 872-4400 or 1-888-939-3333. Fax: (604) 879-9267

Breast Cancer InfoLink, Prairies, Northwest Territories
1331 – 29th Street NW
Calgary, Alberta T2N 4N2
Phone: (403) 670-2113. Fax: (403) 283-1651

Ontario Breast Cancer Information Exchange Project
2075 Bayview Avenue
Toronto, Ontario M4N 3M5
Phone: (416) 480-5899. Fax: (416) 480-6002

Quebec Breast Cancer Information Exchange Network
c/o Hôtel-Dieu de Montréal
3840, rue Saint-Urbain
Montreal, Quebec H2W 1T8
Phone: (514) 843-2930. Fax: (514) 843-2932

THERE ARE MANY local sources of information throughout the country. Call the toll-free Cancer Information Service (1-888-939-3333) for details of sources near where you live. They will also have information about support groups in your area. Or call your local Canadian Cancer Society or Canadian Breast Cancer Foundation chapter.

The Canadian Breast Cancer Network exists to support people affected by breast cancer; they have local representatives in most areas. For the one closest to you, contact the network at: P.O. Box

45115, 2482 Yonge Street, Toronto, Ontario M4P 2H0. Phone: (416) 244-1443. Fax: (416)244-2363.

Look Good . . . Feel Better is a free national program sponsored by the Canadian Cosmetic, Toiletry, and Fragrance Association Foundation, working under the auspices of the Canadian Cancer Society. The program helps women with breast cancer improve their appearance and self-esteem; volunteer cosmetics experts show how to manage treatment-caused appearance changes. Call the Cancer Society for details.

The Internet

INFORMATION ABOUT breast cancer, and access to discussion and news groups, is available on the Internet. There are also several breast cancer news groups. A search for "breast cancer" on the Internet will lead you to the various sources.

If you have an E-mail address, it is easy to have up-to-date information on cancer sent to you. The U.S. National Cancer Institute maintains a free automated mailing system for electronic documents about cancer. To receive a catalog of available documents, send an E-mail message to *cancernet@icicb.nci.nih.gov* with the word *help* in the body of the message. Once you have received and read the catalog, send another message to CancerNet, including the catalog numbers of documents you would like to receive in the body of the message, and you will receive the documents. All the material sent by CancerNet is plain text, which can be loaded into any word processor for formatting and printing.

The Breast Cancer Discussion Group has over 500 subscribers worldwide. You can send an E-mail message to subscribe (*subscribe breast-cancer [your name] to listserv@morgan.ucs.mun.ca*), or contact the list administrator, Dr. Jon Church, who can also be reached by E-mail (*jchurch@morgan.ucs.mun.ca*).

The following publicly accessible sites on the Internet can be reached with net browser software such as Netscape or Internet Explorer:

Breast Cancer Information Center, New York State. Information specific to breast cancer. *nysernet.org/breast/Default.html*

Oncolink, University of Pennsylvania. All cancer types. *cancer.med.upenn.edu/*

Canadian Cancer Society: *www.bc.cancer.ca/ccs/*

B.C. Cancer Agency: *www.bccancer.bc.ca*

Information available on the Internet changes quickly. The Cancer Information Service has up-to-date information on other ways to access help on the Internet.

Videos

Breast Cancer: Management, Treatment and Cure – Part 1: Before Surgery. Pegasus Educational Technologies, 1987.

Echoes of the Sisters: First Nations Women and Breast Cancer. Coyote Collective, First Nations Productions, 1996.

Keeping in Touch. (Breast self-examination teaching video.) Canadian Cancer Society, 1994.

Love, Music and Medicine. Canadian Cancer Society, B.C. and Yukon Division, 1994.

Sharing the Experience: Radiation Therapy for Women with Breast Cancer. B.C. Cancer Agency, Finale Post Productions, Inc., 1994.

The Significant Journey: Breast Cancer Survivors and the Men Who Love Them. American Cancer Society, 1992.

JENNIFER PIKE was born in England and immigrated to Canada as soon as she possibly could. She worked in television and film in both Vancouver and Toronto and did some freelance writing before becoming involved in the book industry about 20 years ago. Currently she is a book seller in Vancouver and underwent her own encounter with breast cancer in 1993.

The publisher would like to dedicate this project to Angie and Annette, and extends thanks to Don Atkins for assistance and support.